UNDERSTANDING
SEXUAL
SATISFACTION

HOW TO GET SEXUAL HEALINGS IN A RELATIONSHIP

Dr. C Conquer

Table Of Contents

Introduction

Sexual Satisfaction

Everyone in a romantic relationship loves having sex, but due to our hectic schedules and busy routines, we often postpone getting involved and engaging in it as supposed.

This is not a healthy action and therefore not recommended at all for love birds.

Disregarding sex and not taking full responsibilities towards having sexual satisfaction is one of the first things that causes resentment and a lack of passion in any relationship.

Sex should always be there in a romantic relationship, regardless of whatever the reasons may be, because it sustains the love, the bond, and makes the relationship lovely and healthy.

Definitions of sexual satisfaction and healings might vary widely depending on individuals involved.

It is generally understood to mean the enjoyment at maximum or climax, enough pleasure one gets from engaging in sexual adventures. Not just having sex.

For most individuals, having a satisfying sexual relationship is crucial but some opt out for reasons beyond their control while some others for reasons best known to them. Some disregard getting sexual healings and satisfaction in their relationships because of ignorance, lack of applicable knowledge and mentorship.

And that's why I am writing this book **"Understanding Sexual Satisfaction"** to showcase **'How To Get Sexual Healings In A Relationship'**

Sexual satisfaction is the reflection of a relationship's happiness, love, commitment, and well-being.

It also regulates the health of relationships, presents opportunities for relationships to be more stable and the chances for breakup or divorce seemingly impossible.

Another aspect of sexual satisfaction is the lasting happiness derived from the quality of the sex one gets from the partner. Healing the soul of every emotionally distressing diseases.

Research indicates that those who struggle to have an orgasm or who suffer from other sexual dysfunctions including erectile dysfunction, premature ejaculation, or others may not think that sexual fulfilment and satisfaction is significant and achievable. Resulting denial of the advantages of sexual satisfaction and emotional healings.
It is well known that having sex makes individuals happier. It also improves relationship quality, fosters more

communication, and heightens emotional connection, among other advantages.

Nevertheless, most sensitive individuals have placed a high value on having a fulfilling sex and feeling satisfied sexually in their relationship.
Therefore, don't disregard sex and start taking full responsibilities towards getting satisfaction from having sex with your romantic partner.
Choosing when and how to have sex is up to you.

Your sexual encounters may be enjoyable and exciting if you are secure, comfortable, and knowledgeable.
It's therefore, very crucial that you know **HOW TO GET SEXUAL SATISFACTION IN A RELATIONSHIP**
Get sexually inspired and enjoy the satisfaction.

Chapter One

Deliberate Connection

Numerous important aspects might influence whether or not a person feels sexually satisfied in a relationship. However, maintaining a deliberate connection through communication is essential to making sure that your demands for intimacy are satisfied.

How to develop a fulfilling sexual connection with your spouse.

1. Give sex top attention.
Sexual activity is essential. There is no doubt that everyone needs it, so make sure your spouse is receiving plenty of it.
Sex always makes a relationship so much better! Ensure that you are scheduling time for it.

Although the unexpectedness and spontaneity of sex are what makes it so enjoyable, it is better to schedule your sex than to not have any at all given the hectic nature of modern living.

It is certainly a turn on when your partner sees how much you want it and how much work you are prepared to put into its fulfilment, so go for it!

2: Talk about sex
Speaking with your spouse about sex is a good idea.
This is what gives your relationship that extra exciting factor.
You should feel comfortable sharing with your spouse what makes you happy during sex and discussing all of your sexual dreams.

How can one in a relationship have sexual satisfaction?
Your sex life would become hotter and more passionate by talking about all of this.

Talk about sex right away if you want your relationship to become stronger!

3. Incorporate some humor

It's possible that boredom or lack of enjoyment in the bedroom is the reason behind your lack of sexual satisfaction in a relationship.

Laughing wildly with your significant other might be the most fulfilling experience ever. It demonstrates your capacity for silliness and stupidity with one another, which demonstrates the strength of your friendship.

It's great for a relationship to crack inside jokes and have sensuous conversations because it releases endorphins and makes you feel pleased and content with your mate.

4. Experience it fully

If you don't feel pleased sexually, what do you do?
You feel every part of it and want to make it better.

Relationships that are sexually fulfilling are dependent on many other factors than just the act of having sex. For example, you need to both like the tension and anticipation of having sex.

The expectation of sex is increased when partners share explicit photos and kiss while the other is at work. It is important to add some spice to the situation since doing so will undoubtedly heighten your desire and want for sexual activity.

5. Beauty lies in imperfection

With the exception of being a sex master or superhero, it is difficult to please your lover every single time. Quit placing so much strain on yourself; instead, project confidence and allow events to unfold naturally. Just be yourself; too cautious and meticulous behavior makes everything fake and dull.

Errors during sex should be very acceptable. It is a strange groan, however, or a humorous remark, since it will only draw you nearer. Try to relax and loosen up a little right then and there, but you can laugh about it afterwards and turn it into an internal joke.

6. Continue to show physical affection
It's not always about sex to keep your lover physically affectionate. It's little gestures of love and devotion like giving them a gentle pat, kissing them, holding their hand, giving them a hug, and making them feel special.

These little gestures of love support the development and maintenance of physical closeness, which enhances sexual satisfaction in a relationship.

7: Negotiate your sexual expectations

Regarding sexual satisfaction, you also need to be really honest about what you require in a sexual relationship. Your significant other cannot read your mind. It's not like they don't want to fulfill your sexual needs and desires, if they don't know what your expectations are, how on earth will they satisfy you?

8: Be honest with what gives you satisfaction

In a romantic relationship, having an honest conversation about your likes, dislikes, and enjoyments might increase sexual happiness.

To be honest means to be open with your partner and be friendly with every aspect of your sexuality. When likes and dislikes are known, certain things will be avoided while some other things will be emphasized to prompt satisfaction.

9: Don't compare your relationship

You may wish to avoid learning how often or how content another couple is with their sexual connection, or how often they have sex.

You will never be pleased with any aspect of your life if you begin comparing it to someone else's, and this also applies to your sexual life.

10. Seek assistance when necessary

If you need assistance, don't be ashamed to ask for it—especially if it will only strengthen your bond. It is important that you get assistance if you need it to ensure that you have a sexually fulfilling relationship due to one or more sexual dysfunctions.

If your marriage or your relationship issues are the cause of your declining sexual pleasure, you could also want assistance in the form of relationship therapy.

Finally

These guidelines for having a fulfilling sexual relationship may seem insignificant and like a waste of time, but believe me when I say they are not.

These principles may completely transform a couple's love life, therefore anybody hoping for a long-lasting, fulfilling relationship should apply them to their everyday lives.

Your romance will rekindle and you two will become closer than before, both physically, spiritually and emotionally if you both decide to deliberately connect with each other.

Deliberately connect and spend quality time together, talk to each other about your sex desires, and you'll be able to see how your relationship's dynamics changes to your favor.

Chapter Two

Help Yourself To Get The Healing And The Satisfaction

Your sexuality is greatly influenced by the changes your body goes through as you age. Sexual issues like erectile dysfunction or vaginal soreness may be brought on by declining hormone levels as well as modifications to neurological and circulatory functioning.

The intensity of early sex may give way to more muted reactions in middle and later life as a result of these physiologic changes. However, the emotional side effects of maturation, such as enhanced self-assurance, improved ability to communicate, and lowered inhibitions, may contribute to the development of a more complex, nuanced, and ultimately fulfilling sexual encounter. But a lot of individuals don't get the full possibility of having sex later in life. Knowing the essential mental and physical components of fulfilling sex can help you deal with the issues more skillfully if they do come up.

Today, treating sexual difficulties is simpler than in the past. If you need to help yourself, expert sex therapists and medications are available. However, you may be able to fix minor sexual problems by changing the way you make love.

Here are a Few Ideas for At-Home Experiments that you can use to Help Yourself Get Sexual Satisfaction and Healings.

1: Learn For Yourself

For every kind of sexual problem, there are a plethora of excellent self-help resources accessible. Look through the Internet or your neighborhood bookshop, choose a few materials that speak to you, and utilize them to educate yourself and your spouse on the issues.

If having a direct conversation is too tough, you and your companion might highlight and show each other the portions you find especially interesting in the healing needed to make your relationship healthy.

2: Take Your Time

Your sexual arousal decreases with age. You may increase your chances of success with your partner by locating a peaceful, cozy, and distraction-free place to have sex. Recognize that it will take longer for you to get aroused and have an orgasm due to the physical changes in your body. If you think about it, having more sex isn't always a bad thing. Incorporating these physical requirements into your routine might lead to new and exciting sexual experiences.

3: Apply Lubricant

Using lubricating liquids and gels, it is often possible to quickly treat the dry vagina that appears during the perimenopause. Use them liberally to steer clear of uncomfortable sexual encounters, which may lead to a waning libido and escalating conflict in relationships.

Talk with your doctor about alternate choices, if lubricants are no longer effective for you, then continue to show physical love.

4: Kissing And Snuggling

Keeping up an emotional and physical relationship requires kissing and snuggling, even when you're worn out, stressed, or angry about some issues, deliberately do the kissing and snuggling. Right!

5: Practice Making Contact

Sex therapists may assist you in re-establishing physical closeness without putting you under strain by using sensate concentration methods. These exercises have several versions seen in self-help books and instructional DVDs.

Asking your spouse to touch you in a way that suits him or her could also be a good idea. This can help you determine how much pressure—from light to heavy—you should apply.

6: Try Assuming Various Postures

Not only can learning various sexual positions make romantic relationships more interesting, but it may also be a useful coping mechanism. For instance, when a guy approaches his partner from behind, the G-spot becomes more stimulated, which may aid in the woman's orgasm.

7: Jot Down Your Dreams

You may use this activity to investigate activities that you and your spouse might find interesting. Try recalling an incident or a movie that made you feel agitated, then tell your spouse about it. Those with low desire will particularly benefit from this.

8: Perform Kegel Exercises

Exercise of the pelvic floor muscles may enhance sexual fitness in both sexes. Tighten the same muscle that you would use to halt pee in midstream to do these exercises.

After two or three seconds of holding the contraction, release it.

Ten times over, repeat.

Aim for five sets each day.

You may do these exercises in a variety of settings, such as a car, a workstation, or a checkout line. Women who want to increase muscular resistance at home may use vaginal weights.

For information on where to get and how to use them, see your physician or a sex therapist.

9: Make An Effort To Unwind

Play a game or go out to a beautiful supper as a relaxing activity to do before having sex. Alternatively, attempt methods of relaxation like yoga or deep breathing exercises.

10: Make Use Of A Vibrator

With the use of this tool, a woman may better understand her sexual reaction and communicate her preferences to her partner.

11: Remain Persistent

Don't give up hope if it seems like nothing you do will work.

Your physician is often in a position to discover the root cause of your sexual issue as well as potential therapies.

He or she could advise you to think about seeing a sex therapist, who can assist you in exploring problems that might be preventing you from having satisfying sex in your relationships.

Chapter Three

Ways To Satisfy Your Sex Partner

In reality, we do not have the natural ability to have amazing sex from the moment we were born.

Recall your first experience of engaging in sexual intimacy with your significant other. It most likely did not cause the earth to tilt on its axis, which is a regular occurrence.

You can gain fantastic sex skills if you're wondering how to make your spouse happy in bed. Let's have some enjoyable sex while learning more about ourselves!

Suggestions for satisfying your sex partner

In the majority of wholesome partnerships, putting your partner's happiness first is essential. It guarantees satisfaction on both ends, giving the couple more reasons to celebrate.

You may use the following strategies to find out how to win over your lover:

1: Evaluate Your Emotional State
First things first: being aware of your feelings and your need for sexual satisfaction.

People often have different desires and wants when it comes to sex, which is an intimate act. Since pleasure is a personal experience, it's important to evaluate how you respond to various actions and simulations.

Understanding your sexual tastes might help you learn how to please your spouse and steer your partner toward actions that satisfy your desires. Your ignorance of yourself may lead to miscommunication and disappointment.

2: Effective Dialogue

Since sexual partners can't read one other's thoughts, chatting a lot is the key to satisfying your spouse. Indeed!

Your partner needs to know what you like and dislike so they can figure out or better still learn how to take you to the seventh heaven of satisfying sex.

It's not necessary to keep your wishes to yourself until you're in bed. Speaking about sex over a romantic meal or cocktail hour may be a great way to initiate foreplay, even if you are unable to follow through on everything you offer.

Don't be afraid to express your feelings to your lover verbally during a passionate kiss, instead of only expressing gratitude with sighs.

Saying things like, "I love it when you touch me there," or "Oh yes, keep doing that," to your partner might help you express exactly what you need from a satisfying sexual encounter.

When you consider pleasing your spouse sexually, are they doing anything that you find unpleasant? Say to them, "Oh, can you focus a little more here and not there?" rather than just shoving away their hand each time and going on to consider how to make your partner happy.

3: Steer Clear Of Routine

You will eventually discover that sex with your spouse that you have developed into a routine—having sex on the same night every week or in the same position every time—is boring.

Change things up and discover how much more sexually fulfilled you are to make sex fantastic again.

If your spouse enjoys engaging in the same sexual activity again and over, how can you win their approval?

Go on impromptu dates, spend Saturday afternoons in bed getting to know each other better, or have sex in the morning before heading to work.

If the kids aren't present, how about in another area of the house?

Consider leaving a few pieces of clothes hanging off your top or skirt to give the impression that you are eager to touch each other.

Try a variety of positions or several positions throughout the evening as you learn how to make love to surprise your lover with some quality time spent together. Does your significant other lead the charge when it comes to making love?

Modify that!

You take the lead, you make the decisions, and you initiate the necessary moves.
They will adore this!

4: Extend The Foreplay

Good sex is more than simply knowing how to please your spouse; it's about making the effort to make the encounter so enjoyable that you get excited thinking about it the next time!

Foreplay is frequently the key to a sexually fulfilled relationship for both men and women.

Make an effort to focus on the foreplay and making it very interesting and enjoyable.
Send each other some flirtatious messages throughout the day to start the foreplay before you get home and prepare for some extraordinary fantastic sex if you know you will be having sex that evening.

If you both inform each other what you intend to do to each other's bodies once you're in bed, you won't have to worry about what happens when a woman or man is not content with the level of sex.

The idea is to prolong the moment of foreplay, whether it's by taking off your clothes piece by piece in the living room or by beginning in the hallway with a shoulder rub and moving your hands to more interesting parts of your partner's body while they're still standing.

5: Message Each Other Before You Meet

Your messages will make it seem as if you are engaged in what the evening has in store, which will increase your urge to meet. There's no need to go straight to the bedroom after you get home.

Do you want to know how to love your spouse more in bed?

Tease one another and let your imaginations run wild until you can get near to one another at last.

6: Don't Be Shy About Having Sex

Making love while using sultry language is quite attractive, particularly to guys. Use terms you are familiar with first if you are hesitant to use particular ones.

If you're wondering how to make your spouse happy in bed, you could assume that talking less and working more is the answer. However, try having some sensual conversations and see the difference.

7: Examine Sex Toys

One excellent tool for achieving sexual fulfilment is a sex toy.

A growing number of couples are including them in their sex play for really fulfilling sex now that they are widely available.

Look at a catalogue or website jointly if you're thinking "How to keep my husband or wife sexually satisfied."
Tell each other what you think would be good to try and why you are drawn to that particular item above others.

In addition to what your spouse is currently doing during sex, looking together through various toys is a terrific method to let your partner know your preferences and what you will need to send you into an orgasm.

8: Talk About Your Dreams

It might be challenging to please your partner if they are not open to trying new things. It's a difficult job, to be sure, but it's not impossible to push someone over their comfort zone.

Communicating your desires to your spouse is another approach to learning how to be more sexually intimate.

You may boost your partner's libido and sexual happiness by discussing your dreams with them and listening to theirs.

Recall that fantasies are just that—fantasies. It doesn't follow that they or you would want to carry out these actions in the actual world.
Telling each other what you dream about when you think about excellent sex is part of the sexiness of it, even if it will never really happen.

9: Use GGG

Do you know what the abbreviation GGG stands for?
It represents Generosity, Goodness, and Games.
Being GGG should be your objective if you want to satiate and satisfy each other sexually.

You look forward to your private times with your spouse, like sex, and are excellent in bed.

Giving in bed is being considerate of your partner's enjoyment and being generous.

The game indicates you're willing to try new things and to listen to your partner's requests and recommendations for a fulfilling, seductive, and thrilling sexual life.

At least once, be open to trying new things—as long as you feel safe doing so. You never know when that "one thing" may turn you on so much that it will start to happen often throughout your romantic encounters.

Having good sex is not complicated. To be present, break up the routine with surprises, and look outside the box (and the bed!), all it takes is two people. That's it!

If you're still unsure about how to win a guy over, try implementing these suggestions gradually and observe the results.

10: Avoid Being Complacent

Do you want to know how to make your spouse happy?

Make sure you appreciate what you have and strive every day to make things more interesting and thrilling.

It's important to avoid becoming comfortable with your shared sexual happiness since this might cause issues down the road.

It's important to continuously re-evaluate what works for you and your partner since your preferences for sexual activity may vary over time.

Finally

You're already heading in the correct direction if you're thinking about ways to appease your partner.

Making an effort to find more engaging methods for your spouse to have sex will help prevent your relationship from fizzling out.

Assess your sexual tastes and be upfront with your spouse about it. Try new things and pay attention to your partner's sexual arousal when they share it with you.

You may improve the quality of your marriage and the pleasure your spouse gets sexually by learning, listening, and growing as a couple.

Chapter Four

Features Linked To Greater Sexual Satisfaction

A happy love and romantic relationship will to a large extent depend on sexual satisfaction to triumph.

Sexual satisfaction between the love birds most often do lead to greater levels of love, commitment, and stability in the love relationship.

Regretfully, sexual dysfunctions, or issues with sex, are not uncommon.

According to research, 10%–50% of men and 25%–60% of women in the US have some sort of sexual dysfunction, which often manifests as a lack of desire for sex or trouble having an orgasm.

Sexual pleasure versus dysfunction is significantly influenced by age, physical health, and mental well-being.

As women age and as long as lubrication is not a problem, they often have increased sexual performance, but males tend to experience greater erectile dysfunction. However because oestrogen plays a part in lubrication and drops in women after menopause, lubrication may become problematic if left untreated.

The typical drop in arousal that happens during the first trimester of pregnancy, with recovery generally occurring during the later two trimesters, provides another illustration of the probable role that hormones play in female sexual pleasure.

Measurement of sexual satisfaction

Adults in committed relationships, such as marriage, often perform better sexually than single adults, and persons with greater educational attainment usually have better sexual lives than adults with lower educational attainment. Although there doesn't seem to be much of a correlation between race and ethnicity and the overall prevalence of sexual dysfunction, there seems to be some variation in the kind of dysfunction depending on this group. For instance, compared to Hispanic and Caucasian women, African-American women often exhibit lower levels of sexual desire, whereas Caucasian women seem to feel greater physical discomfort during intercourse.

Sexually charged life events, such as experiencing physical or sexual abuse, tend to impair women's ability to perform sexually; however, same-sex relationships or more than five-lifetime partners do not. Although having sex more often is generally linked to a marriage with conventional gender roles, the degree of enjoyment in such relationships has not been well-researched.

Features linked to greater sexual satisfaction in females

Women's sexual pleasure is influenced by several things.

High levels of sexual desire and contentment with one's profession and love relationship all contribute to sexual pleasure, while ageing may often work against it.

Sexually pleased women often exhibit levels of desire that are very similar to those of their partners.

There is evidence to suggest that penis width may be a more significant predictor of sexual pleasure than penile length.

Sexual satisfaction is also more common among women who self-stimulate.

The argument there is that women who self-stimulate are more conscious of their sexual urges and demands.

It is often believed that communication—both in general and about one's sexual needs—is the most important element in obtaining sexual happiness.
In comparison to their nonassertive counterparts, women who exhibit high degrees of sexual assertiveness also tend to have greater levels of desire, orgasm capacity, and sexual pleasure.

Couples tend to have greater levels of sexual pleasure the more often they show love toward one another, both romantically and non-sexually.
It's interesting to note that sexual pleasure might be influenced by communication style. For instance, it's believed that nonverbal communication during sex is more likely to be linked to sexual pleasure than vocal communication.

Women and their partners would be well advised to protect their emotional and physical health, be affectionate in all aspects of their relationships, become aware of their own sexual needs, and express those needs to their partners openly and courteously, given the significance of sexual satisfaction in maintaining health and happiness, as well as the multiple factors involved in female sexual satisfaction.

Health Benefits of Sex
Sex has many benefits outside of the bedroom.

Did you know that having sex is healthy for you in addition to being enjoyable?
It is accurate.
Sex has many health advantages, including reducing stress, heart attack, and cancer risks.
Intimacy and connecting with your spouse are facilitated by sex.
Not only does this sense of closeness make you feel good, but it also lowers anxiety and improves your general health.

Which would you prefer—better sleep or a more robust immune system?

Actions between the laps may help you obtain all of this and more.

1. Reduce colds and strengthen your immune system

Sick days decrease with more sex.

Results from research comparing sexually active and non-active individuals indicate as much.

Your body produces more antibodies to fight against viruses, bacteria, and other microorganisms that cause common diseases when you have sex.

Naturally, maintaining a strong immune system involves more than just having happy relationships.

Maintaining current vaccines, eating a balanced diet, exercising, getting enough sleep, and maintaining good health are all factors in building robust defences against infectious diseases.

2. Increase your sexual attraction

Unbelievably, having sex is the greatest way to boost a declining libido!

Having sex increases desire.

Additionally, having sex may help address discomfort and vaginal dryness, which can make it difficult for some women to engage in sexual activity.

Improved vaginal lubrication, increased vaginal blood flow, and increased tissue flexibility are all brought on by sex and contribute to enhanced desire and better, more enjoyable sex.

3. Boost the bladder control

About 30% of women will have urinary incontinence at some time in their lives.

A woman's pelvic floor muscles are strengthened and toned when she has frequent orgasms. The same muscles that women employ for Kegel exercises are also activated during orgasms.

Stronger pelvic muscles reduce the chance of mishaps and urinal leaks.

4. Reduce your blood pressure

Do you have high blood pressure as millions of other people do?

You may reduce it with sex.

Numerous studies have shown a connection between reduced systolic blood pressure—the initial reading on a blood pressure test—and sexual activity in particular, not masturbation.

This is encouraging news for anyone seeking a simple addition to a healthy lifestyle (diet, exercise, stress management), as well as prescription treatments, to lower their blood pressure. While they can't completely replace blood pressure medications, sex sessions may be a helpful supplement.

5. Sex qualifies as exercise

Sex expels calories just as any other kind of physical exercise does!

A minute of TV viewing while seated burns around one calorie.

Sex works a variety of muscle groups and raises the heart rate, burning around 5 calories every minute. While regular sex cannot take the place of workouts, having an active, healthy sexual life is a pleasant approach to increasing your physical activity intake.

6. Reduce the risk of heart attacks

Desire a healthier heart?

Increase your sex.

Hormone levels, such as those of oestrogen and testosterone, are regulated by sexual activity.

Osteoporosis and heart disease may occur when these hormones are out of balance. More is better when it comes to safeguarding heart health via sexual activity. Men who engaged in at least two sexual encounters each week had a 50% lower risk of dying from heart disease compared to their less promiscuous counterparts, according to research.

7. Sex reduces pain

Orgasm and sexual stimulation, including masturbation, may help numb pain.

Both exercises may raise your pain threshold and lessen your perception of pain.

Hormones that may help inhibit pain signals are released during orgasms.

Some women claim that masturbating as a kind of self-stimulation helps lessen headache, arthritic, and menstrual cramp symptoms.

8. Sex may lower the risk of prostate cancer

Other health advantages of sex are exclusive to men.

According to one research, males who ejaculated frequently—defined as at least 21 times per month—had a lower risk of prostate cancer than those who did not.

It made no difference whether the ejaculations were from sex, masturbation, or midnight burps. Of course, ejaculation frequency is not the only factor that affects prostate cancer risk, but this was an intriguing discovery.

9. Sex boosts your sleep
You may have better sleep with sex.
This is because orgasm mimics the natural sleep-inducing hormone prolactin's release. Prolactin promotes sensations of contentment and drowsiness.
This is only one of the many explanations for why you may find it easier to fall asleep after a sexual encounter.

10. Sex reduces stress
It is quite therapeutic to have sex.
This is because physical contact, affection, sex, and emotional attachment generate the production of "feel-good" chemicals that foster harmony and connection.
Substances that activate the brain's reward and pleasure systems are also released during sexual stimulation.

Building closeness and connection may improve general health and reduce anxiety.

11. Sex burns calorie

Sex is another activity that burns calories. According to one research, having sex burns over 108 calories per thirty minutes in young men and women!

That is sufficient to burn 3,570 calories in 32 half-hour sessions, which is slightly more than the amount of calories in one pound.

12. Sex boosts your heart health

The bedroom might hold the key to improved cardiovascular health.

Science indicates that physical effort during sexual activity does not increase the risk of stroke, despite what some individuals may fear.

Over 900 men participated in a 20-year trial, and the results showed that having sex often did not raise the risk of stroke.

They discovered that sex protects against deadly heart attacks, too.

Compared to men who had sex fewer than once a month, men who had sex at least twice a week had a 50% lower chance of a fatal heart attack.

13. Sex boosts your health and wellness

People are social beings by nature.

Your general health and well-being are improved when you interact with friends and relatives.

Having close relationships with others, especially your spouse, makes you happier and healthier than those with fewer ties. Research backs this up, seriously!

14. Sex boost closeness and bonds in relationships

Warm, close connections may be developed by giving and receiving hugs and cuddles. Couples connect via the production of oxytocin, a hormone that is stimulated by sex and orgasms.

This so-called "love hormone" contributes to the development of trust and love.

In research involving women who were not yet menopausal, the more time the women spent cuddling and holding their partners, the greater the amounts of oxytocin in their bodies.

The hormone also promotes kindness and warm emotions.

15. Sex makes you appear more youthful

Forget about anti-aging lotions and surgery—having sex also keeps you appearing younger.

Frequent intercourse promotes the production of testosterone and oestrogen, two hormones that help you seem youthful and energetic.

Oestrogen improves younger-looking skin and glossy hair.

In one research, judges estimated the ages of participants by looking at them via a one-way mirror.

Individuals who engaged in sexual activity with a regular partner at least four times a week were thought to be seven to twelve years younger than their true age.

16. Sex makes you live longer

How can one live a longer life?

Perhaps it's getting more sex.

Those who had the most orgasms had half the mortality risk compared to those who did not ejaculate regularly in ten-year research including over one thousand middle-aged males.

Longevity is influenced by a variety of circumstances, but one simple and enjoyable approach to increasing your age may be to have an active sexual life.

17. Sex increases intelligence

Having sex indeed has advantages for the whole body.

Having frequent sex may improve brain function.

Researchers discovered that having sex causes the brain to shift into a more analytical thinking and processing state. Additionally, research on animals suggests that sex improves memory-related brain regions.

18. Fertilization is easier with sex

As far as growing a family is concerned, practice makes perfect.

Men who ejaculated every day for a week produced better-quality sperm than those who did not, according to fertility clinic research. Sperm from the males who ejaculated daily contained less fragmented DNA than the sperm from the men who ejaculated less often.

Healthy DNA is implied by less broken DNA.

Furthermore, healthy DNA-containing robust sperm have a higher chance of fertilizing an egg.

When Rise In Temperature Affects Sexual Urge And Satisfaction

1: Put on light clothing

When temperature affects your mode for sexual arousal, kindly switch from heavy clothes to lighten clothings.

What works best are absorbent, lightweight, and loose-fitting textiles like cotton.

Just use one layer.

Additionally, choose light coloured clothes, since darker ones have the ability to absorb heat and intensify your heat.

2: Select the proper mattress

The ideal materials for your bedding are cotton or linen, which will allow for enough airflow, keep you cool, and wicks away perspiration.

Blends of polyester and cotton won't keep you as dry and cool.

Next, search for a "thread count" between 200 and 400. If it's higher, the cloth may retain more heat and moisture and won't breathe as effectively.

3: Put your bed sheets in the chill

Simply place them back on your bed after a few minutes in the freezer. You may put them in the refrigerator if that's too chilly. Use an airtight plastic bag to keep them away from food, liquids, and ice. It won't stay cold all night, but it could be warm enough for you to get some sleep.

4: Have a cool shower

It also works to just sponge off with cold water or take a bath.

It ought to aid in bodily cooling.

Additionally, warm water helps you cool down since it causes your skin and hair to evaporate. However, try not to overheat the restroom. That can exacerbate the situation.

5: Warm, frozen water bottle

In the winter, do you bring a "hot water bottle" to bed to stay warm? Yes, it may also be used as a cooling tool.

Simply place it in the freezer after filling it with water. Before using it, you may need to cover it with a cloth to protect your skin.

Additionally, you might save any buckwheat pillows or packs that you typically use in the freezer or refrigerator to reheat during the cooler months.

6: Change the air

If you have air conditioning, that's your best option.

Just lower the temperature when you start to feel overheated.

If that isn't an option, you may use one, two, or three fans to get the air circulating.

Create a passage for the air via open windows.

For an even stronger cooling boost, place an oven-roasting pan full of ice cubes in front of the fan.

7: Put it in ice

You might use an ice pack if you're too heated. Or soak a towel with cold water and apply it on "pulse points" like your wrists, ankles, the crooks of your elbows, and the backs of your knees.

Just be sure to protect your skin by covering it with a towel, and limit the amount of time you do it to 20 minutes.

8: Put on sunscreen.

Your body will have a tougher time cooling down if you get sunburned and get dehydrated. When you're outdoors, particularly in the direct sunlight, wear sunglasses and a wide-brimmed hat.

And apply sunscreen to any exposed skin. Apply sunscreen with a minimum SPF of 30 minutes before venturing outdoors.
You will need to reapply throughout the day if you want to remain outside.

9: Take it easy

Don't get right into a lot of activity, particularly outside exercise, if you find yourself in a suddenly hot new area.
Give it a two-week trial before stepping up the exercise level.
Lift your legs over your head and lie down if you feel dizzy.
As soon as you can, try to find a cool place to be and start drinking water.

10: Keep an eye on the caffeine

That's the "stimulant" in your coffee in the morning that gets you motivated and out the door.
For the most part, it's harmless, although it might cause your body temperature to rise.

You may not want that if you're already feeling warm.

It's not limited to coffee either.

It may also be found in many over-the-counter medications, chocolate, tea, sodas, and sports beverages.

Examine the package to be certain.

11: Don't drink

If you're frying in the heat, an ice-cold beer or drink could seem like the perfect solution.

However, alcohol can lower your core temperature while making you feel even warmer.

If you're already overheated, this is not a healthy mix and might leave you queasy and lightheaded.

In addition, excessive alcohol use may disrupt your hormone balance, leading to transient increases in body temperature known as "hot flashes."

12: Switch out the beds

A sleeping buddy can keep you warm throughout the cold.

But you could think about your bed if you're having trouble staying cool throughout the summer.

You may even try to find a room with more windows or one that is lower down in the home since these would be cooler.

A decent, chilly night's sleep will make you feel better the following day, even if you may miss your sleeping mate.

13: Cool with water

Your body uses sweat as an air conditioner, and for it to function correctly, it requires water.

In terms of sports, it is crucial.

A few hours before you go for physical activity, fill up your tank with a few drinks.

Take a water bottle with you to practices or games, and aim to sip from it around every fifteen minutes or so.

Recall that if you're in the air conditioning or pool, you may not notice the perspiration you lose.

Chapter Five

Is She Sexually Satisfied?

A fulfilling sexual life is essential to every successful relationship.

The emotional and psychological bond between couples is equally as important as the actual physical act.

A woman's sexual satisfaction might be a strong sign that the relationship is succeeding.

So how can you tell whether your significant other is happy?

The significance of sexual satisfaction in a relationship

Let's first explore the significance of sexual happiness in a relationship before moving on to the indications.

It has been shown that having sex may strengthen emotional bonds, lessen stress and anxiety, and increase general well-being.

It's critical to have open lines of communication and regular check-ins with your spouse in a relationship to make sure that both of you are content and contented. Couples may improve closeness and strengthen their bond by concentrating on sexual satisfaction.

Additionally, having a fulfilling sexual life might benefit one's physical well-being.
Frequent intercourse has been associated with lowered blood pressure, a better immune system, and a decreased risk of heart disease.
It may also raise self-esteem and enhance the quality of sleep.
As a result, giving priority to sexual satisfaction in a relationship offers possible health advantages in addition to improving the emotional bond between couples.

How to interpret your partner's intimate body language

Body language may convey more information about sexual fulfilment than words alone.

Be mindful of subliminal indicators such as heaving, labored breathing, and elevated heart rate.

These signals may suggest that your significant other is taking pleasure in your work. However, if they seem tight, uninterested, or inattentive, it could be time to adjust the situation or follow up to find out if there are any worries or problems.

Paying attention to your partner's facial expressions is another crucial component in interpreting their body language in the bedroom.

When they grin or display a happy expression, it's obvious they're having fun. To make sure everything is well, it's crucial to stop and speak with them if they seem uncomfortable or in pain.

It's also important to keep in mind that each individual has a unique body language, so what one person may interpret as a sign of enjoyment may not translate the same way for another.

In every sexual experience, communication is essential, so don't be scared to find out what your partner enjoys and dislikes. By doing so, you can make sure that the encounter is enjoyable for both of you and have a greater understanding of their body language.

The significance of communication in attaining sexual satisfaction

In every relationship, communication is essential, but it's more important in intimate ones.

Discuss your likes and dislikes with your spouse, and urge them to do the same. Understanding one another's wants and requirements allows you to cooperate towards getting a mutually satisfying outcome.

Talking honestly and openly with each other might strengthen your bond.
Don't be frightened to do so.

Consent is a crucial component of communication in attaining sexual enjoyment.
It is essential to communicate your comfort level and discomfort levels clearly and consistently.
Using protection, talking about limits, and checking in with each other during sex are all examples of this.
Always provide passionate, unreserved consent that is appreciated by both parties.
Additionally, talking things out might assist in resolving any problems or worries that can come up in the bedroom.
It's important to communicate and work together to find a solution if something isn't working for you or your spouse.
This might include experimenting, investigating various methods, or, if necessary, obtaining expert assistance.

You and your partner may have a safe and fulfilling sexual encounter if you communicate honestly and freely.

Investigating the relationship between sexual satisfaction and emotional intimacy

Sexual pleasure and emotional connection often go hand in hand.

In any relationship built on mutual respect, trust, and open communication, partners are more likely to feel secure and at ease in bed.

Beyond just having sex, intimacy is the state of being both physically and emotionally connected to your spouse.

Couples that prioritize emotional connection will definitely have more rewarding sexual satisfaction in their romantic relationship.

Studies have shown that couples who place a high value on emotional connection are more likely to report feeling more satisfied with their sexual life.

This is so that couples may be more honest and vulnerable with one another as emotional closeness fosters a feeling of safety and security.

A more satisfying sexual encounter results from couples communicating their wants and wishes more often when they feel emotionally connected.

Furthermore, emotional closeness may strengthen the emotional connection between couples, resulting in a more robust and fulfilling relationship overall.

Advice for increasing your partner's sexual satisfaction

Enhancing sexual pleasure in a relationship may be done in a variety of ways. Experiment with various sex postures and sex gadgets in your privacy with your partner.

Prioritize intimacy daily and make time for enjoying it.

Outside of the bedroom, express your love and gratitude to your mate; this will build emotional and trusting bonds.

Keep in mind that having a fulfilling sexual relationship involves more than just the physical act; it also involves an emotional and psychological bond.

Communication is a key component in enhancing sexual happiness in a relationship.

It's important to communicate with your spouse honestly about your needs, limits, and any worries you may have. This may promote mutual respect and a sense of being heard, which can help couples better comprehend one another's sexual needs.

A guide to satisfying your partner through an understanding of female orgasm

Knowing how to have an orgasm is one of the keys to satisfying a woman's sexual needs.

Here, communication is essential.

Women differ tremendously in their bodies and desires, so ***find out*** from your spouse how they want to be caressed or aroused.

Recall that the goal ought to be to create a welcoming and secure atmosphere.

Not all orgasms are the ultimate aim; sometimes, the trip itself is just as fulfilling.

It's crucial to remember that having a sexual climax is not the only way to feel pleasure. Women are capable of receiving pleasure from a wide range of sources, including vaginal, clitoral, and even non-genital stimulation.

A more satisfying sexual encounter might result from experimenting with various forms of touch and discovering what feels good for both parties.

It's also critical to realize that not all women can have an orgasm only via penetrating intercourse.

For many women, experiencing an orgasm requires clitoral stimulation.

For this reason, you must talk to your spouse and experiment with various forms of stimulation and touch to determine what suits you both the best.

How to establish a comfortable and safe space for sexual exploration

Although it might be scary to explore new sexual avenues, it's crucial to provide a welcoming and secure space for this kind of activity.

Take things gently and talk to your spouse about what they feel comfortable with.

Be mindful of each other's personal space and only proceed with things that both of you feel comfortable with.

Establishing a safe phrase or signal that either partner may use to express discomfort or the desire to stop is also crucial.

In the process of sexual exploration, this might assist in avoiding any miscommunications or misunderstandings.

Before starting any new activities, be sure to discuss any worries or anxieties you may have honestly and openly.

Setting the atmosphere with elements like lighting, music, or even fragrances may help create a cozy space.

Try out several combinations to see what suits you and your partner the best.

Recall that the intention is to provide a space where both parties feel valued, comfortable, and free to explore their sexuality without constraints or criticism.

Stress and anxiety's effects on sexual satisfaction

One's ability to enjoy sexuality might suffer greatly from stress. Making time for intimacy may be challenging when one or both partners are experiencing stress or anxiety.

Make self-care a priority and find methods to unwind with your partner.

Think about using alternative methods to develop closeness, including snuggling or having a bath together.

Recall that closeness may take many other forms and that having sex is not the only way to feel satisfied sexually.

It's crucial to remember that physical arousal and desire may be impacted by stress and worry.

It may be challenging to experience sexual arousal while the body is under stress. This may increase frustration and make the problem worse.

It's important to discuss your feelings with your spouse and collaborate to find answers. In some situations, getting expert assistance could be required.

You and your spouse may work through any underlying problems that could be causing tension and worry with the assistance of a therapist. They may also provide methods and strategies for reducing stress and enhancing sex enjoyment.

Recall that asking for assistance may result in a happier, better relationship and is a display of strength.

Frequently held myths regarding female sexual satisfaction and strategies for dispelling them

Many myths exist about female sexual pleasure, one of which is the idea that women don't find sex to be as enjoyable as men do.

These ideas have the potential to be damaging and undermine a woman's confidence in her sexuality.

It's critical to dispel these myths and foster a healthy sense of self-worth about sexual fulfilment.

These myths may be dispelled and a more satisfying sexual life can result from self-discovery and communication with your spouse.

Another widespread misperception about female sexual pleasure is that penetrative intercourse is the only way to get it.

This misconception may be restricted as it disregards other sexually pleasurable activities including oral sex, manual stimulation, and the use of sex toys.

Prioritizing reciprocal pleasure and satisfaction.
It's important to investigate and discuss what feels good and what doesn't with your spouse.
We can make sexual experiences more inclusive and satisfying for all participants if we expand our conception of what sexual fulfilment is.

The advantages of trying out various sexual positions and methods

To increase sexual pleasure, it may be entertaining and exhilarating to experiment with various sexual positions and approaches.
Take things one step at a time and be honest and transparent with your spouse about what you want to do.
Take creative liberties and enjoy examining each other's bodies.

Experimenting with various sexual positions and methods may enhance one's overall sexual health as well as one's level of sexual happiness.

Couples may avoid boredom in the bedroom and break free from sex rituals by experimenting.

Furthermore, experimenting with various postures and methods may assist partners in learning what their bodies respond to and pave the way for future, more satisfying sex.

How to handle problems with incompatibility in the bedroom

Partners may sometimes discover that their sexual requirements or preferences are different.

It's critical to have an amicable and transparent conversation about these incompatibilities.

It's important to communicate and work together to identify a middle ground that suits both sides.

While some trial, error and compromise may be necessary, reaching mutual satisfaction should always be the aim.

It's also important to keep in mind that sexual compatibility varies throughout time. It's possible that what formerly worked for both parties is no longer effective.
It's critical to keep lines of communication open and to re-evaluate what each partner needs and desires in the bedroom.
This may maintain the relationship happy and healthy by preventing any resentment or irritation from growing.

The significance of vulnerability and trust in reaching sexual satisfaction
Finally, the key to having a satisfying sexual relationship is vulnerability and trust. Partners are more inclined to let their guard down and enjoy the moment to the fullest when they feel comfortable and safe in each other's company.

Deeper degrees of intimacy and fulfilment may be experienced by couples via the development of trust and the creation of a trustworthy environment.

In general, a good relationship must include sexual satisfaction.

These indicators might help you better understand your partner's wants and goals so you can collaborate to get a mutually satisfying outcome.

Never forget that communication is essential, therefore don't be scared to discuss your sexual wants and wishes with your spouse honestly and openly.

It's crucial to remember that vulnerability and trust may be hard to build, particularly if there have been previous traumas or trust concerns.

Partners must collaborate to provide a secure and encouraging space where each party may freely communicate their wants and goals.

To address any underlying problems that could be impeding the growth of trust and vulnerability in the relationship, this may include going through treatment or counselling.

Chapter Six

Strategies To Maintain Intimacy And Satisfaction

Sexual arousal, ecstasy, gratification, and pleasure do not have to fade with age.

Over time, there is a reduction in sexual desire and happiness in many relationships. Put otherwise, matrimony is difficult. However, research results are averages, meaning that some couples do not see a drop in sexual pleasure and passion with time.

If properly nourished, sexual desire may last for decades within a marriage, according to recent studies.

When around 39,000 US adults who had been dating for three years or more were asked what sustains their sexual desire, these patterns emerged:

1. Mood establishment

Increased sexual pleasure, arousal, and passion may result from setting the tone for sex in a married relationship.

During the day, send your spouse a seductive SMS.

Additionally, allocate time for foreplay, which includes soft, leisurely kissing that may progress to firm kissing that may intensify desire and sexual excitement.

A weekend away at a cabin or hotel may provide plenty of alone time for a couple, much like a honeymoon.

You may create an environment in your marriage where there is plenty of sexual desire and happiness.

2. Diverse sexual orientations

Sometimes, a sexual narrative that begins and ends with sexual activity is taught via popular media.

For husband and wife to have long-lasting sexual passion and fulfilment, however, some variation is necessary.

Some ways to add variation to the relationship are to wear lingerie, massage, discuss and act out sexual fantasies, engage in genital clutching, and slow down during sex.

Before doing anything new, however, make sure you discuss sexual diversity with your partner.

Before putting methods into effect, both spouses should approve of them. Take into account various approaches, utilize your imagination, and put into effect what benefits both partners.

3. Dialog

Sexual communication that is non-verbal and verbal are the two primary forms of communication that enhance sexual enjoyment.

Does having a sexual conversation or making nonverbal cues about sex increase sexual satisfaction?

I could be asking the incorrect question.

Studies have shown that the most crucial factor in communication is not the mode of communication used. What counts is if a couple is content with the kind of sex communication they have.

Think about sharing information on your sexual preferences, including your likes, dislikes, wants, and frequency of sex.

Various topics regarding sex in marriage may come up when talking about preferences.

Couples talk about sexual inconsistencies or issues sometimes, and sometimes they talk about their preferences.

Married couples need to understand one another, so having these discussions about sex is normal and should not be scary. Communicating allows partners to better attend to their sexual impulses and comprehend what the other wants in the bedroom.

4. Aim outside

Other data suggests that turning outward in sex is related to the three themes of what drives sexual desire and fulfilment.

Turning outward to tend to a spouse's needs can literally double your sexual pleasure: You get satisfaction not only from your sexual response but from your partner's as well, love and concern for one's partner shifts the focus away from the self in a sexual relationship and toward the other person.

Strangely, both men and women are considerably more likely to have sexual fulfilment when they approach sex with this unselfish attitude.

Sexual desire and fulfilment may last as long as both partners project an external image and work to make the other feel happy.

5. Willingness

In conclusion, a married couple's level of sexual passion and pleasure does not have to wane with time.

Nonetheless, couples need to be deliberate in addition to these four crucial concepts. Finding time and energy for sex in a marriage may be challenging due to a variety of factors, including work obligations, children's extracurricular activities, exercise, home chores, errands, and many more.

Sexual closeness may still lose priority over some of these other aspects even if couples follow all four of the aforementioned advice if they are not deliberate.

Here, intentionality refers to the continuous scheduling of intimate sexual activities.

By sexual communication, sexual diversity, mood-setting, and turning outward, one may intentionally and persistently maintain sexual desire.

Couples may have more sexual pleasure and passion by making this deliberate and consistent effort.

Chapter Seven

How Long Is Too Long To Go Without Sex?

Since every person's relationship is diverse and complicated, every couple will have various relationship challenges.

However, spending extended periods without having sex is a frequent issue that many couples encounter.

Partners may have difficulties with their sex life, or more precisely, the absence of it if there is improper communication and a lack of clarity on expectations.

Although discussing sex might be awkward for some, if sex ceases in a relationship and these gaps are not cleared up via talk, it can lead to pain and uncertainty.

Why does my relationship no longer involve sex?

Significant declines in sex in a romantic relationship may result from somethings that undermines confidence problems with body image and shape.

An increase in negative self-thoughts and partner-thoughts.

Anxiety and overanalyzing.

increased levels of tension.

Ineffective communication.

A diminished sense of intimacy with one's spouse.

Overall discontent with the relationship.

It might be challenging for you to discuss your thoughts and sexual happiness with your spouse.

In addition to being unpleasant, this lack of conversation may heighten general unhappiness.

How much time does relationship dry spells last?

Many clients in solo or couples therapy who report that they are going through a dry spell and have not had any intimate sexual interaction often went through some months without having any kind of sexual contact.

However, this is something that varies in relationships, person-specific and should not be universally applied.

Numerous factors may directly alter how long a partner is sexually absent from a relationship.

A "dry spell" may be ended quickly, for instance, by improving the quality of acts of service, emotional closeness, or communication.

A dry period might resolve faster even if you only talk about it and acknowledge the sexual absence and its causes.

Is it normal to skip sex for a few months?

As previously said, a lot of treatment clients report that they are going through a dry period and have not had any sexual activity for some months.

This is particular to each individual and relationship rather than something that can be readily generalized.

This time frame suggests that although going some months without having sex is not inherently abnormal, going six months or more without having sex may be a general indicator of relationship problems. Every relationship, however, is different, and as such, each will have its expectations on when and how frequently sexual activity should occur.

If you skip too much sexual activity

Not having sex may lead to several serious psychological and physical issues that can affect one's relationships with others as well as oneself.

Long stretches without sex can psychologically damage a committed sexual relationship by making both partners feel hurt or rejected. It can also drastically reduce their levels of intimacy and connectedness, especially if they choose to ignore or avoid discussing the problem.

Scientific research has shown that having sex physically lowers stress and cortisol levels, reduces inflammation, elevates mood, and balances hormone activity throughout the body.

Lack of sex may be a contributing factor to any of the dysregulations mentioned above, even if it may not necessarily be the primary cause.

But not having sex doesn't usually mean that you should worry too much.

While it's acceptable to crave sex or physical pleasure, many individuals also have reasonable feelings of not wanting it or even being averse to it.

Hormonal fluctuations, poor libido, or even being naturally asexual or demisexual—as is the case for many—can all contribute to this. Even while having sex may be reviving and improving your connection with a partner, not everyone finds that having sex is essential to having a happy and fulfilling life.

What are the things that indicates lack of sexual activity?

The causes of some couples' sex cessation seem to be very comparable to the consequences of non-sex.

Whether they are the reason or the result of an undesired absence of sex in a relationship, these problems almost often accompany it.

The following are just a few examples of the behavioral and emotional indicators of a lack of sexual activity in a relationship:

1- Intolerance.

2- A rise in distrust.

3- Issues with body image.

4- Bad ideas about oneself and one's relationship.

5- Concern and moping.

6- Elevated levels of stress.

7- A decline in the level of communication.

8- A reduction in the general sense of closeness that one feels.

9- Overall discontent with the relationship.

This is not to argue that a happy, healthy, and communicative relationship cannot exist without sex.

But, sex may be a significant and essential component of love relationships, and the absence of the understanding and relief it can provide might indicate—or even initiate—issues with emotional strain, communication, and even a certain level of mistrust.

Can a relationship be ruined by absence of sex?

A lack of sex in a romantic relationship may be a sign of general relational health issues, even if it may not be the exact cause of the breakup.

The regularity and consistency of sexual activity in romantic relationships may serve as a reliable gauge of the partners' overall emotions of happiness, emotional closeness, and connectivity.

As a useful tool for assessing the health of a relationship, it may provide therapists working with couples with a window into the relationship.

Sexual conduct tends to be more fulfilling and frequent in relationships that are in better health.

What is the ideal frequency of sex for a couple?

The optimal frequency of sexual activity for a couple depends on their particular relationship and should include their respective sexual arousal levels and wants, as well as the practical times of the week when they can have sex.

The easiest method to gauge how often you should be seeing your partner for sex is to ask yourself, "How often does it make me feel sexually fulfilled and satisfied?" What frequency fulfils my partner's sexual desires?

Although this varies from couple to couple, many couples find that having sex at least once a week satisfies their physical and emotional requirements.

Despite the popular perception that sexual activity should be impulsive, it is perfectly acceptable and often wise to schedule dates based on each person's availability.

Instead of assuming that the other person and themselves agree, this may assist each party in clearly communicating their expectations and goals.

Does a relationship need to involve sex?

Without having sex, a relationship is possible.

As was previously said, some people identify as asexual, which means they have no interest in or desire for sexual behavior. Asexuals participate completely in the romantic aspects of relationships, but they are generally not at all attracted to sex. Asexuality is a spectrum condition; individuals who identify as asexual may still choose to engage in sexual relations with partners, while others may have no interest in engaging in any kind of sexual activity.

It is possible for a brief, healthy break from sexual activity to continue if all participants in the relationship do not identify as asexual, but it has to be addressed and agreed upon by both.

It is never advisable to withhold sex from your spouse to manipulate them; this is generally seen as abusive conduct.

How Much Time Is Too Much Without a Partner?

Everybody probably has a different idea of how long they think it is "too long" to stay single.

These explanations most likely also stem from the individual's values, beliefs, and conceptions of what their relationships and life ought to be like.

Rather than pondering the length of time that might be too lengthy to go without a relationship, consider the following:

What motivates me to look for a new relationship?

Are these motivations or wants ones that I can take care of on my own, or do I require the assistance of a social support system?

Do I still need time to recover from that relationship?

How will I know or be able to tell whether I'm ready to start dating again?

What restrictions do I have on a possible romantic relationship?

This justification is entirely subjective, but individuals who wait a while to start a new relationship usually need that time to recover and turn their attention inside, no matter how long that may take.

Ultimately, for many individuals, having sex is an exciting and significant aspect of life. But whether it's a step back from intimacy or back into having sex, communication, and understanding are essential to ensuring that the transition is a healthy and thoughtful one when sex vanishes from a love partnership.

Chapter Eight

Good Habits Of Couples That Achieves Sexual Satisfaction

They Give A Broad Definition of Sex
Sexually content couples often realize that having sex isn't the only aspect of their relationship and satisfaction.

Research also reveals that they often have at least one personal encounter every week.

A set routine isn't a guarantee of happiness right away.

Physical intimacy, however, is often an indication that a relationship between a couple is healthy.

They Acquire Education
Sexual pleasure may be equated with knowledge.

You may have the best possible sex life by getting to know each other's bodily erotic zones, what makes you turn on, and how much stimulation you require.

Their Touch

The establishment of connection and trust may be facilitated by physical touch.

Using a method called sensate concentration, sex therapists treat patients. This activity investigates the sensations evoked by various forms of contact.

A sexual "goal" like an orgasm or penetration is also lessened, which relieves pressure.

Partners might get closer and enjoy intimacy more when they engage in sensual touch practices.

They Put Their Trust in One Another

Empirical research indicates that dissatisfaction is more common among couples who lie about their preferences for certain activities in the bedroom.

Thus, if you are having problems experiencing an orgasm or your desire is lacking, let each other know.

Inform your partner if you are uncomfortable with something or if you feel self-conscious about your body.

They Consult with Therapists

By assisting you with touch exercises, teaching you about arousal and desire, and improving your communication skills, sessions with a licensed sex therapist may ease intimate concerns.

Talk therapy may also be beneficial to your relationship as a whole if your troubles are the result of other concerns.

They continue to be Adaptable

Sexuality lacks a normal.

Each person has a particular set of preferences, frequency of want, and importance of the item.

The stresses of everyday life, ageing, and physical health may all have an impact on your libido and priorities.

A more satisfying sex life may be attained by couples who have an open mind and are flexible about their sex requirements.

This improves their self-esteem.

They Produce Time

Your physical response to sexual stimulation slows down as you get older.

Having and maintaining an erection might be more difficult in older men due to lower testosterone levels.

Women who have dry vaginas and delayed arousal may experience a reduction in oestrogen after menopause.

Aim to provide enough time for each other to enjoy sex.

They Make Experiments

Can there be a rut in your sexual life?

To resurrect the spice, experiment with various postures, motions, touches, and stimulations.

To experience climaxes more often, the new procedures could potentially intensify feelings.

They Attend to Their mates.

It has been shown by research that happy couples are those who prioritize their partner's satisfaction and who enjoy each other's company.

This can include playing out your partner's sexual fantasies or having sex more often or at different times than usual.

People Look for Approval

It takes practice to become perfect: any action that makes you happy, such as physical activity, laughing, sex, or creating art, increases the feel-good endorphins in your body and strengthens the response pathway that makes you feel aroused more readily.

They Employ Instruments

Some may see it as an admission that they need assistance to prick their partners or see nothing wrong with using lubricant to relieve dryness or supporting their posture with a cushion during intercourse.

It is, however, the reverse.

You will have a better experience if you pay more attention to both your partner's and your comfort.

They Execute It

Although it could seem depressing.

Better intimate relationships are experienced by couples who feel that putting in effort and hard work—rather than searching for their soulmate—is the key to a fulfilling sexual life.

They Ban Pornography

For some couples, erotica in books or photographs may put a spark in the bedroom. However, some men's capacity to get an erection and have an orgasm with their spouse may be hindered by a strong pornographic habit.

A further false impression of what real-life sex is like is created by porn.

That might damage the relationship and erode their partner's sense of self.

Orgasm is Not An Obsession For Them

Not every sexual experience aims to reach a climax.

It may put a great deal of strain on some relationships.

Closeness may be developed just by sensually touching or connecting in any manner that suits both of you.

They converse with one another.

Achieving pleasurable sex may greatly benefit from knowing where your partner's sexual "starting point" is.

Some people—men mostly—can instantaneously and unprompted get into the mood they want.

Others need a trigger to get aroused, most often women.

Your mutual happiness might increase if you accept such differences.

Chapter Nine

Positions For Satisfying Sex

While many sex positions satisfy both parties, the finest ones are those that you and your partner can enjoy together.
Have you given different styles a try?
Changing up your posture in bed might assist you achieve orgasm by increasing stimulation.

Sexual activity is a pursuit of unlimited variation.
Couples may enjoy hundreds of steamy sex positions that bring the bodies of men and women together for pleasure.
Being aware of different sex positions might make you a more creative and better lover for your spouse if you're in a straight relationship.

Which Ways Make the Best Sexual Experiences for Both Parties?

Every relationship has a different response to it.

Testing various sex positions offers an opportunity to bring different ways of experiencing pleasure into sexual intimacy and a sexual relationship.

I would define the best position as the position that works best for the individual or individuals involved.

Eating the same meal every day for twenty years does not guarantee that you will be happiest with it.

All you're receiving are the nutrients. However, you may find that the dish tastes different and becomes more interesting if you try adding a little amount of parsley to it.

Changing roles in a relationship might have that effect.

There are other nonphysical aspects to take into account.

Consider intimacy as an example.

Intimacy may result in greater sexual experiences for many individuals, particularly women since partners feel secure and trusted enough to explore new things and ask for what they want.

Reasons to Experiment with Different Sexual Positions

We know that this has been a stressful period and that can make it hard to get aroused and stay aroused.

Experimenting might increase your level of arousal.

Trying new things can help you find what works for your body and your relationship, which will benefit you for the rest of your life.

These manoeuvres don't need you to be a gymnast to be successful.

To increase the amount of heat and sexual satisfaction between the sexual partners, consider novel sex positions rather than "crazy sex positions."

Not every position is for everyone, and that's okay.
However, it doesn't mean you shouldn't attempt new and different things, even if the positions listed here don't work for you (maybe you've already tried them).
One of the things that draws us in and keeps us coming back for more is novelty.
We tend to lose interest in sex when it is the same every time.
Changing up our postures might be a convenient method to inject some freshness and originality into our sexual lives.

1: The Missionary Role or In-Person
Intimate but not always fulfilling on both sides

The lady is in a basic sex position, lying on her back with her legs apart and her knees slightly bent.

The male uses his arms or elbows to support his body weight while he lays between her legs and inserts his penis into her vagina.

The issue with this sexual role is that it does not provide women with the same level of pleasure as the missionary role does.

In this posture, the man's pelvis may occasionally excite the clitoris and provide a great deal of intimacy via direct facial contact.

However, the penis's angle prevents deep penetration or stimulation of the G-spot, which is sensed through the vagina's front wall and is thought by some specialists to be a trigger for female orgasms.

In addition, several women lament that there is insufficient clitoral stimulation in this sex position to produce climax.

Using a different sex position might be a crucial step in "closing the orgasm gap" if the most popular one isn't providing women with regular orgasms.

Put differently, don't restrict oneself to the role of missionary.

The greatest ways for both parties to gain from having hot, fulfilling intercourse

Try some of these female-friendly poses if you want to improve the sex you have and spice up your encounters.

Many provide couples the opportunity for clitoral stimulation, which 36.6 percent of women said they required during sexual activity in order to have an orgasm.

2: Top Woman or Cowgirl
Sensations and penetration depth vary; clitoral stimulation.

The lady faces the guy while he is on his back, kneeling, straddling his pelvis, and guiding his penis into her vagina.
Then she may lay on him or sit up.

This is a great position for a woman to control the depth of penetration.
The woman has the power to decide how much of his penis she wants when she is in charge.
Additionally, it's a great location for getting different kinds of stimulation.
The woman's nipples may contract while her torso is upright, which may cause increased arousal.
Having access to the clitoris for stimulation is beneficial.
Additionally, the lady has the option to grind, bounce, or create hip circles; each produces a somewhat distinct feeling.
Men who are very susceptible to visual stimuli may lay back and observe the female partner, adding, "This is also a good position for a person with a penis if they have back

issues because it's almost a resting position for them,"

3: Reverse Rider on Top or Reverse Cowgirl

Playing with the buttocks, stimulating the eyes, creating chances for diversity; may cause discomfort

The lady sits astride her spouse, facing her feet, and slides the penis into her vagina as the guy sleeps on his back on the bed.

The thrusts' cadence and rhythm are within the woman's control.

As he gets to see his partner's back and buttocks, the penetrating partner may find this position particularly arousing.

Grabbing or squeezing the buttocks might improve the encounter for both parties.

As the woman must sit up straight or lean back to fit the angle of the penis, this position may be challenging to get right.

If you're leaning forward, it can be painful and uncomfortable for the man because it could almost feel like his penis is breaking.

You have your partner bend his knees and then brace yourself by placing your hands on his thighs, on pillows on either side of him, or behind you.

This may be one of those positions that is better in theory than in practice.

You might want to grind on his penis as a foreplay position before you start having sex.

4: Tailored Design or Back Entry

G-spot stimulation, deep penetration, although posture may seem impersonal

The lady is on all fours in this posture, using her hands and knees to support herself. The guy ducks under her and reaches inside her vagina.

The optimal sexual position for the vagina is this one.

The guy is free to caress a large portion of the woman's body and to push his pelvis quickly and forcefully.

Additionally, the posture permits effective G-spot stimulation.

Switch It Up: Some women argue that the lack of in-person interaction makes this sex position excessively impersonal. "Move your knees closer to your chest and arch your back so your partner can lean into you near your face and you can make eye contact if you want closer eye contact with this position.

5: The Screw

Deep, strong penetration.

The lady leans forward and lays on the edge of the bed, her forearm and hip supporting her while her lover enters her vagina from behind.

For a more firm grip on the penis, the lady might keep her thighs together.

However, if she spreads her legs, a guy will push from behind and expose her clitoris for caresses.

This may be a more comfortable and easier position, but you're still getting that deeper penetration like doggy style.

Switch It Up, your spouse may readily bend down to make out with you and the clitoris is easily accessible.

6: Side by Side or In a Sideways Position

Closeness and deep eye contact.

The lady and the guy are facing each other while lying on their sides.

In order for the guy to implant his penis, the lady raises her upper leg.

The leg may then be crossed over his leg or wrapped around his waist.

This position is ideal for morning sex when you may be a bit tired.

You are in close proximity to your partner's face, which provides a great deal of intimacy.

When making love, the couple might kiss and caress one another.

The sex position is calming, doesn't demand much energy from either partner, and provides excellent clitoral stimulation.

Switch It Up, if a lady crosses both of her legs over her partner's waist, penetration will be enhanced.
This gives you excellent access to the clitoris, which you may stimulate with a toy or your finger.
I believe that everyone is in a terrific position with this.
It also provides the coziness of snuggling.

7: Lazy Dog or Flat Iron
Tightness at entrance, strong stimulation
The lady is face down on the bed, her hips slightly lifted and her legs straight.
Her lover penetrates her vagina from behind (you may do this by placing a cushion under your hips).
The woman's legs will be closer together while she is on her stomach, which will

accommodate her partner's penis more snugly.

This may result in a brand-new, stronger feeling.

This is a really good way to increase the penetrating partner's experience of tightness. Because the partner may offer dual stimulation by reaching around with his hand or a sex toy, it's also beneficial for clitoral stimulation.

Additionally, since you're angling your body such that your penis is perfectly aligned to stroke against the G-spot, it's a wonderful posture for G-spot stimulation.

8: Face-to-Face

This might be a more intensified missionary position with significant eye contact and clitoral stimulation.

The lady comes into his lap, face to face, and wraps her legs behind him while the guy sits on the edge of the bed or in a comfortable sitting posture.

The lady has control over how quickly she thrusts.

Intimacy may be increased by this position's facilitation of direct clitoral stimulation and eye contact.

You can touch and caress your partner's body almost wherever you like since your hands are free.

This is a really impactful position for people who are aroused with eye contact.

Similar to a missionary, except you interact with people directly.

By putting his hands on her hips, her partner may move her up and down, which relieves some of the strain on the vaginal donor.

9: Dip in Pretzels

Deep penetration that may cause G-spot activation.

The male straddles the woman's right leg while she rests on her right side.

After that, the guy enters his vagina by pulling his partner's left leg up and around his left side.

Intimacy and thorough penetration are both made possible by this posture, which permits eye contact.

Change It Up, to obtain a deeper angle, you can also take your left leg and pull it toward your chest.

Your hands will be free, so you may run them over each other's bodies.

And you have amazing access to the clitoris for both partners.

This position — depending on your angle — can also offer G-spot stimulation.

10: The Coital Alignment Technique, or CAT,

Coastal Stimulation.

Roll with CAT if you'd rather rock than shove.

The primary distinction between this position and the missionary position is that the guy presses his penis' base into the clitoris, bringing the two sections of his body into touch.

When they do, the pair keeps their eyes on each other and rocks back and forth.

This is a slightly different way of having sex. Instead of pushing, you sway back and forth. As a result of the continuous stimulation, this lengthens the man's sex and raises the possibility that a woman may have an orgasm.

We have a tendency to be very goal-oriented in our daily lives.

As soon as we wake up in the morning, we have to hurry to get out the door, get breakfast, and go to work. It causes a great deal of strain and stress in both our bodies and thoughts.

Many folks believe that having sex has become just another thing they must do. However, sexual partners have to be really in love and enjoy each other's company. Changing places might be a great way to reignite that relationship.

So, attempting something new may be enjoyable, satisfying and beneficial.

Chapter Ten

Explorable Sex Positions

Top Sexual Positions

Searching for the greatest possible position to have satisfying sex? You've arrived at the ideal location.

Compiled here is a list of several enjoyable sexual positions, ranging from well-known and comforting options to creative new concepts you've never tried.

Some of the actions in this list will definitely surprise you.

However, I promise that none of these roles are so unconventional that it will be uncomfortable to propose them to your significant other.

Broadly Available

Adopt a flat back position. Place your legs around your partner's waist while they kneel on the edge of the bed with their knees slightly apart. Next, arch your back to elevate your hips and pelvis. While they do the thrusting, have your partner support you by grabbing the small of your back.

X Indicates the Location

Put your legs up and either maintain them straight or place your feet on your partner's chest for a unique take on the missionary pose. The X section enters at the shins, where you cross your legs to provide a tighter fit and more friction.

The Position 69

This is challenging the traditional shared oral sex position. While the other person supports them, one person stands erect and the other does a handstand. This should enable you to get to each other's private parts; however, you may need to end it quickly to avoid having too much blood flow to your brain. Actually, this may be more of a "just to say we did it" type of role.

The 69 without

Just mutual oral sex will do in this feel-good sex position—no penetration required. For the 69th slot, either partner may be at the top or bottom. All you need to do is arrange yourselves head to toe so that you may make love to each other at the same time.

The Screw

Your lover enters you from behind as you lay on your side on the edge of the bed, butt facing out. For optimal experience, keep your legs tightly together (for both of you). To save your partner from having to perform all the effort, you may also shove backward.

The bouncy chair

First, instruct your spouse to kneel. As they kneel, place the balls of their feet on the floor and their butts on their heels. With your feet flat on the floor on each side of their legs, face them and straddle their lap.

To manage the rhythm and penetration after you're in position and their penis or strap-on is within you, bounce on the balls of your feet. The personal time will be delightful because of the near closeness.

Tigress

Imagine a variation on reverse cowgirling. Lay your partner down on the floor, then sit on top of them with your back to them. Put one hand on their chest and reach back now. As you raise and lower yourself, use your hand for stability. This gives you total control over the penetration depth and pace. If you discover that you need a lift, you may also ask them to place their hands around your waist.

The extra benefit? It will certainly help that you can glance back and see people staring at you.

The Pretzel

It will take some manoeuvring to get this one, but it will be well worth the effort. To begin, lie on the bed with your lover kneeling over you so that their legs are straddling your hips. Next, draw one leg across your body and then in toward your chest. Your lower body should be twisted, similar to a calming twist at the conclusion of a yoga practice, but your back should remain rest flat on the bed. Your spouse should be using their chest or stomach to brace your leg. Your lover may enter you with deep, pleasurable thrusts from this position, and the sideways angle really jiggles things up for novel and thrilling experiences.

Elevated Wheelbarrow

This one is simple for committed yogis, but it will send a surge of blood straight up your spine. After you're in downward dog, softly lift up your legs and wrap them over your partner's waist. In addition to using your arms to support you, they will also hold you up by your hips.

Wheelbarrow in a seated position

The modified sitting wheelbarrow is an option if the standing wheelbarrow seems like too much arm effort. Place your companion on the edge of the sofa or bed in this posture. It's much simpler to wrap your legs over their waist after assuming downward dog since you can rest your lower body on the bed instead of bearing your whole weight.

Friends in Fitness

One leg is lifted while you lay on your side, and your spouse balances your ankle on their shoulder while sitting on their knees, straddling your lower leg, and penetrating you.

The Spider

Do you recall executing the crab walk during a creative exercise session, or maybe it was during a gym class? The two partners meet in the centre while in the crab walking position. You should be within their legs with both of yours. Raise your pelvis to place yourself on top of your partner while you're in the lead. You are in charge of the rocking from there.

The Inverted Pyramid

Sometimes it's better to keep things simple. As your spouse penetrates you with a finger or sex object, lay on your back and let them do the same to you. What an overachiever.

The Lotus

The Lotus position is a time-tested but effective way to add some spice to any situation, even if some adaptability is required, the result is well worth it. The technique is as follows: Cross your legs while you lie on your back. Now have your spouse get on top of you while you bring your crossed legs as near to your chest as you can. Try to stay in the crossed-legged posture for as long as possible. Though it's a massive hip opener, the angle is perfect for a G-spot orgasm.

Naughty Tee

Place your spouse on their side with their back to the top of the bed to begin working on a new alphabet letter. After that, choose a position that is perpendicular to them, move your hips to meet theirs, bend your knees, and lay flat on the bed with your feet behind your partner's butt. On the bed, your bodies make a T shape together. Your lover may shove into you from this posture.

Crouching Dragon, Standing Tiger

This little twist makes for much hotter behind-the-back sex. Let your standing partner enter you from behind while you are kneeling on the bed, sofa, dining table, floor, or any other raised surface. Compared to if you were just hunched over, this enables them to strike numerous angles.

Depending on how far apart you lay your legs, the experience may vary. Experiment with different leg openings to see what feels most comfortable for you.

The Churn of Butter

This one offers the perfect position if you want to have a great stretch during your next sex session! As you hold your back with your hands, have your partner enter you with his penis as you lie on your back with your legs over your head and your butt up, much to a backward roll.

The Love of Oneself

For this one, one item is required: a mirror. With their back to the mirror, your companion takes a chair. Seated on their knees, you sneak peeks at the sensual spectacle that unfolds before you.

The Intersection, also known as The Hashtag

After all, it's a pound symbol (get it?). To get into the position, lie on your side with your partner kneeling in front of you and raising your upper leg, forming a scissors posture.

The X iPhone

The notion that greater is better is celebrated by this action. As you maintain your head and neck on the bed and rely on your shoulders for support, raise your hips into a bridge position while lying on your back. Your spouse holds your hips up while straddling you on the bed. It's undoubtedly an improvement over your typical schedule, but if anything goes wrong, don't contact tech support.

Ice and Fire

Go take a shower and cover your significant other's body with warm water. Next, give them an oral treatment by melting an ice cube in your mouth. A fantastic transition into spectacular shower sex, the combination of your chilly tongue and the hot water spraying all over their body will be mind-blowing.

Cowgirl

This position is a timeless classic that gives you power over your companion. Most likely, you are already familiar with the basic technique: have your partner lay down, straddle them, and ride them toward the horizon. The best thing about this specific posture is that it gives the top partner complete control over the rhythm's depth and tempo. It's also among the greatest positions for pregnant sex because of how easy it is to move.

Cowgirl Bending Forward

For unmatched stimulation to your G-spot, fold forward while in the cowgirl pose. Grind your body over your partner's while kissing, caressing, and maybe even romancing their hair, as opposed to bouncing up and down.

Cowgirl Astride, also known as Cowgirl Leaning Back

Here's another entertaining sex pose inspired by cowgirl. As usual, climb to the top, but this time, bend backward and place your hands on your partner's knees. They may grip your buttocks for more stability. You'll experience maximal G-spot stimulation once again at this angle. The added benefit of having easy access to the clit is this position.

Inverted Cowgirl

How about we switch up the classic cowgirl pose? Everything remains the same, except now you'll be facing their feet instead of their head. This allows for extra-deep penetration while maintaining control over the angle and tempo that work best for your body.

The Twerk

The reverse cowgirl is enhanced by the twerk. Lean forward and take on the reverse cowgirl pose, placing your arms on their thighs. Then all you have to do to have sex is arch your back and rock back and forth while popping your booty up and down, like you're twerking.

AKA The Scoop, The Spoon

This is the ideal way to enjoy a treat in the morning. Turning to your spouse, spooning them, and going down is all it takes to get from a deep slumber to morning sex. First, each couple lies on their side. When the "big spoon" comes in from behind, the "little spoon" may tuck their knees in little.

The Sticky Spoon

Put yourself in the spoon pose, but raise one leg! You may either take up the position on the sofa (where you can then hang your foot over the back rest) or prop it up with pillows.

In a Doggy Way

In a list of the greatest sex positions, it would be negligent if I did not include doggie style. With your partner standing behind you, get on all fours. You may grip onto your waist or hips and let your partner push, or you can grind it out from this position.

LeapFrog, also known as Froggy-Style

Instead of remaining in a tabletop posture, you will adopt a doggie style where you rest your head on your forearms and your forearms on the bed. This position allows you to easily touch yourself as your partner thrusts, much like in doggie style.

The Lazy Dog, also known as The Flatiron

In this instance, one partner enters the other from the behind, much like a dog. However, the receiving partner should just lay on their stomach with their legs straight back behind them, as opposed to kneeling. This results in a snug fit that feels fantastic for both parties.

Pressing the Cushion

A sofa and a vibrator are needed for this enjoyable sexual posture. Sit on the sofa in the traditional dog posture, with the receiving partner facing the back of the couch. Position a vibrator behind the pillow and press it up to your vagina. When your lover enters you from behind, the vibrator will arouse your clitoris and make the whole cushion come to life. It sounds wonderful, doesn't it?

Breaking Up Bamboo

You know how sometimes getting into your chaps and riding around the bedroom is the last thing you want to do after a stressful day?

Cowgirls, you may relax; this sex position is on your side. Assume missionary position by first laying on your back and having your partner climb on top of you. Next, lift one leg and place it against their head, resting it on their shoulder. Maintain the other leg extended on the bed. Penetration with penis will feel much deeper when done with one leg up. Ask them to kneel instead if you're uncomfortable, if your hamstrings aren't as flexible as you thought they would be to avoid overstretching your elevated leg.

The Devil

The Anvil sex positions are trustworthy for a purpose. As in the missionary position, lie on your back and let your lover straddle you. Raise your legs so they rest on your partner's chest, neck, or shoulders as opposed to keeping them down. What was the outcome? maintaining eye contact and the closeness of a face-to-face posture while executing deeper thrusts and a tighter fit.

Falling Water

After lying down on the bed, your partner should slide backward such that their upper body is at an angle over the bed and onto the floor. After your partner is in position, straddle and ride them while they attempt to contain their blood flow. You may even switch places and experience the adrenaline for yourself.

The Om

Have your companion get on board by sitting cross-legged. For tantric-style sex, wrap your legs around their waist and rock back and forth. You may make eye contact with your partner in this face-to-face posture, which makes it quite intimate.

The Yum Yam

With one minor exception, this is identical to the om. The spouse in the top position should bend back and support themselves with their hands after attaining the om posture. Though that's a fantastic angle both visually and sensationally, you most likely won't be able to hold it for very long. But even if you just spend a little while doing it, it will be well worth it.

The head of the committee

Locate a chair that doesn't have arms and force your spouse to sit in their undies. After that, sit on their lap with your back to them and guide their hand to the area of your body that you want to be touched. Reposition yourself such that they are inside of you while you're still sitting on them until you can no longer stand the taunting. As you move back and forth, encourage them to continue caressing you until you both feel fulfilled.

The Room with Champagne

There's one little, but noticeable, difference between this and the chairwoman: keep your legs folded and your knees together rather than straddling your spouse. This keeps everything very tight and creates a whole distinct experience.

The aquatic

Position your butt so that it is parallel to the edge of the bed or table; if you want more height, lay a cushion under your hips. After that, raise your legs straight up into the air, calf-to-tail like a mermaid. A finger or penis, may be used by the inserting partner to enter.

The Reverse Spoon or The Reverse Scoop, Side by Side

Both of you lay on your sides in this sex position. With the exception of facing each other, it's exactly like the spooning position. Starting in a missionary fashion, you may gradually shift onto your sides without losing contact with one another. Both partners have equal control over the thrust depth in this position.

The Octopus

Positioning yourself between your partner's wide legs while lying on your back, you can see that they are sitting upright. Draw yourself nearer to them, cross your legs over their shoulders, and let them to suck into you. Proceed to gently push it away from there. However, proceed cautiously, since it is simple for the strap-on or penis to come loose in this posture.

The Sitter

In essence, this is face-sitting light. As would occur in a face-sitting posture, the person having oral sex straddles the provider and lowers themselves into their mouth; however, the receiver then leans forward and uses their hands to support themselves. This allows the donor unrestricted access from underneath while also giving them additional breathing space.

The Wizard of Pinball

The Pinball Wizard is one of our favorite titles for sexual positions. It entails laying on your back and raising your hips to a bridge posture (keeping your shoulders on the bed). From a kneeling posture, your partner may support your hips while they enter you.

The Cross

Place your feet at the foot of the bed and your head close to the pillows while lying on your stomach. To allow the penetrating partner to enter you from behind, have them lay on their stomach perpendicular to your body.

The graduating student

It's time to let go! Place yourself in the missionary position first, then fully extend your legs. Holding your legs out in a V shape with your hands (you may grab your ankles or calves) can help you keep them open.

The Shell

Although it calls for much greater flexibility, this role is remarkably similar to that of valedictorian. You tuck your feet behind your head rather than extending your legs into a V. Maximum stimulation is possible as a result of vulva and clitoris exposure being maximized.

The Method of Coital Alignment

Sex therapists advise you to adopt this posture to maximize your chances of experiencing an orgasm during sexual activity. Once you're in the missionary position, your partner moves to the top of the bed, positioning their chest to about where your shoulders are. Once they are as near to you as possible, they should put their weight on you and rock back and forth until their pubic bone grinds on your clitoris. It's okay if you don't orgasm with this motion alone, but it will be simpler if you use a clitoral toy like Eva or a cock ring!

The Inverse Missionary

For those who can pull it off, sex stances like this one may be surprisingly enjoyable. However, it does need some flexibility. Assume a supine position on your back, with your partner's head pointing in the direction of your feet. For balance, they'll probably have to be on their hands and knees. Then, they will push in and out as normal, most likely with little thrusts to keep you both where you are. If your spouse appreciates anal stimulation, you may use your fingers to give them the stimulation you want. You can also hold their butt to assist position them the way you want. (We can even suggest anal vibrators and other anal sex toys.)

The Chair for Relaxation

Place yourself on top of your spouse, facing them, and then recline backwards, as if you were lounging in a lounge chair, with your hands resting on the bed or your partner's legs. From this point on, you and your partner may push each other or you can take a pause and let your partner play with your clit. Even if your penis or dildo isn't moving, sometimes having it inside of you increases clitoral pleasure.

Additionally, you will get the most G-spot stimulation when reclining backward because of the angle that is created.

Traditional Missionary

It's not necessary to try out new sex positions all the time to enjoy yourself in bed. A tried-and-true classic may function well in certain situations. similar to a missionary, even though society insists on making missionary work seem bland, it often prevails in the feel-good category. The bottom is very hot! Feeling someone's body pressing on you, making you both sweat profusely, and keeping eye contact?

Chapter Eleven

Food That Can Help To Avoid Premature Ejaculation

Do you know that at least one in three men between the ages of 18 and 59 experience premature ejaculation (PE) at some point in their lives?

Yes, You heard it right!.

With changing lifestyles, and the significant increase in stress levels, this problem is going to disturb the males more aggressively in the coming days.

But the question is what can we do to avoid PE?

The answer is multifold, including lifestyle changes, stress management, and proper nutrition.

In this book, we are going to focus on micro nutrition that can be obtained from certain foods that we should plan to include in our daily eating habits.

Start these foods early in your life and you will be able to keep the PE away for a long time.

However, please note that if you are already suffering from PE, the food alone may not be able to extend quick and sufficient help. You may need to have additional supplements.

So without wasting any more time, let's dig deep and know how and what food helps you fight PE.

Food That Can Help To Avoid Premature Ejaculation

Consuming a balanced diet that includes foods rich in nutrients like zinc, magnesium, and omega-3 fatty acids can potentially help avoid premature ejaculation by promoting overall sexual health and enhancing control during sexual activity.

Additionally, certain foods, such as fruits, vegetables, and whole grains, can contribute to improved cardiovascular health, which is linked to better blood circulation and stamina in the bedroom.

While there isn't a specific diet proven to treat premature ejaculation, certain foods are believed to have potential benefits for sexual health.

Keep in mind that individual responses vary, and it's important to consult with a healthcare professional for personalized advice.

Here are some foods that are commonly associated with promoting overall sexual health, so let's have a look at some dietary recommendations to help address premature ejaculation:

1. Green onion

Green onions are aphrodisiacs that will increase the stamina and power to perform sexual activities and aid in PE management. Take a crushed green onion and mix it in water three times a day until you regain your stamina and interest.

2. Carrots

Carrots are a nutrient-rich vegetable that provides various essential vitamins and minerals. Here are some key nutrients found in carrots:

Vitamin A: Carrots are particularly rich in beta-carotene, a precursor to vitamin A, which is essential for vision, immune function, and skin health.

Vitamin K1: Important for blood clotting and bone health.

Vitamin C: An antioxidant that supports the immune system, skin health, and aids in the absorption of iron from plant-based foods.

Potassium: Helps regulate blood pressure and fluid balance in the body.

Fiber: Contributes to digestive health and helps maintain a feeling of fullness.

Biotin: Supports healthy skin, hair, and nails.

Vitamin B6: Involved in various enzymatic reactions in the body, including the metabolism of amino acids.

Folate (Vitamin B9): Important for cell division and the formation of DNA.

Manganese: A trace mineral involved in bone formation, blood clotting, and reducing inflammation.

Copper: Essential for the formation of red blood cells and the absorption of iron.

Eating a variety of nutrient-dense foods, including carrots, contributes to a balanced and healthy diet.

Premature ejaculation can have various causes, including psychological, hormonal, or neurological factors. It's important to approach any claims about the effectiveness of specific foods with a critical mindset.

3. Banana
High in potassium and vitamin B, bananas are thought to aid in the production of hormones essential for sexual health.

4. Ladyfinger 'Okra'
Ladyfinger is a nutritious vegetable, rich in vitamins, minerals, and fiber.
Some people believe that the ingredients in okra may enhance overall health and potentially impact sexual activities positively.
Specific claims about its effectiveness in addressing premature ejaculation are not yet well-established in scientific literature.

5. Ginger & Honey

Both ginger and honey have been used in traditional medicine for various health purposes, but their specific effects on sexual function are not well-established.

Ginger is known for its anti-inflammatory and antioxidant properties, while honey is often praised for its potential antibacterial and immune-boosting properties. Some people believe that the combination of these two ingredients may enhance overall health and potentially impact sexual function positively.

6. Garlic

Garlic does contain allicin, a compound with antioxidant and anti-inflammatory properties. Some believe that these properties may have positive effects on overall cardiovascular health, which can indirectly impact sexual function by improving blood flow.

7. Eggs

Eggs are a nutrient-rich food that provides several vitamins and minerals that play a role in overall health, including aspects that may influence sexual performance.
Here are some nutrients in eggs and their potential contributions:

Protein: Eggs are a good source of high-quality protein, which is essential for the body's overall functioning, including the repair and maintenance of tissues.

Vitamin B12: This vitamin is crucial for nerve function and the production of red blood cells, which can indirectly impact energy levels and overall vitality.

Vitamin D: Important for bone health and potentially linked to testosterone levels, although the relationship is complex and varies among individuals.

Zinc: This mineral is involved in the production of testosterone and may contribute to reproductive health.

Choline: Essential for the production of acetylcholine, a neurotransmitter that plays a role in sexual arousal.

While these nutrients are important for overall health, it's crucial to emphasize that no single food can guarantee improved sexual performance.

8. Watermelon

Watermelon contains an amino acid called citrulline, which is converted into arginine in the body.
Arginine is known to have vasodilatory effects, meaning it can relax blood vessels and improve blood flow.

Improved blood flow can have positive effects on overall cardiovascular health, including the blood flow to the genital area.

Some people believe that this enhanced blood flow may have benefits for sexual function.

9. Dark Chocolate.
Contains phenylethylamine, a compound that can promote a sense of well-being and potentially enhance libido.

10. Asparagus
Rich in vitamin B, asparagus is believed to boost arousal and help regulate hormones.

11. Almonds
Almonds are a nutrient-rich food that can contribute to overall health, including sexual health, due to the presence of certain vitamins and minerals.

Almonds are a good source of vitamin E, zinc, and magnesium, which play roles in reproductive health.

Vitamin E, for example, is an antioxidant that may support overall cardiovascular health.
Magnesium and zinc are essential minerals that contribute to various bodily functions, including hormone regulation.

Maintaining a balanced diet that includes a variety of nutrient-rich foods can positively impact overall well-being and sexual participation.

12. Mushrooms
Some traditional medicine practices and anecdotal reports suggest that certain mushrooms, like Cordyceps or Reishi, have potential benefits for sexual health and overall well-being.

Cordyceps, for example, is believed by some to have adaptogenic properties that could help manage stress, which may contribute to improvements in sexual function.

Reishi mushrooms are often associated with immune system support and overall vitality.

It's important to note that while these mushrooms have been used in traditional medicine, scientific research on their efficacy in treating premature ejaculation specifically is limited.

13. Walnuts

Rich in omega-3 fatty acids, walnuts may support overall sexual function and sperm health.

14. Avocado

Packed with healthy fats and vitamin E, avocados contribute to better blood circulation and overall cardiovascular health that improves sexual performance.

15. Coffee

While there is some anecdotal evidence suggesting that caffeine, found in coffee, may have certain positive effects on sexual performance, there is limited scientific support for coffee as a remedy for premature ejaculation.

Caffeine is a stimulant that can increase alertness and improve blood flow, which might contribute to increased sexual performance. However, it's important to note that excessive caffeine intake can lead to negative effects such as increased anxiety or insomnia, which could potentially impact sexual function negatively.

16. Pumpkin Seeds

High in zinc, pumpkin seeds are associated with testosterone production and may have positive effects on sexual health.

17. Oysters

Known for their zinc content, oysters may play a role in testosterone production and overall sexual health.

Incorporating these foods into your diet can be a natural and holistic way to avoid PE by addressing various contributing factors, including blood flow, hormone levels, stamina, and overall sexual health.

However, please do note that the dietary changes are to avoid PE and not to solve the PE.

If you are already impacted by PE and have started observing it very recently, you should try these foods for 2-3 months.

You should get some positive results but these may not be what you are looking for.

Because foods are effective in prevention and cure requires something more.

There is a high probability that you may need to go for some supplements for 3-6 months and once you solve the problem up to your satisfaction levels, you can return to foods that are effective preventive tools.

Finally, Premature ejaculation can take a toll on your relationship with your partner. But the right preventive approach at the right time can keep you away from the risk of PE.

Your diet plays a vital role in keeping you sexually active. It's essential to maintain a balanced and varied diet for overall well-being.
Adding the above foods to your eating habits is a good preventive measure.
Additionally, lifestyle factors such as regular exercise, stress management, and open communication with your partner are crucial for a healthy sexual relationship.

However, if You are already impacted by PE, you need some additional supplements.
If premature ejaculation is a concern, consulting with a good healthcare professional or a sex therapist is advisable for personalized guidance and potential treatments.

Chapter Twelve

Ways To Postpone Ejaculation

Ejaculation
Ejaculation is the release of semen from the penis, typically accompanied by orgasm. It is a physiological process that occurs during sexual arousal and climax.

Ejaculation involves a series of muscular contractions and the expulsion of seminal fluid, which contains sperm, from the male reproductive system.

The process is controlled by the central nervous system, and it involves the coordination of various muscles, including those in the pelvic area.

Ejaculation serves a reproductive function, delivering sperm from the male reproductive tract into the female reproductive tract during sexual intercourse, allowing for the potential fertilization of an egg.

While ejaculation is a normal part of the male sexual response, issues related to ejaculation, such as premature ejaculation or delayed ejaculation, can occur and may be a source of concern for some individuals. If someone has specific concerns or questions about ejaculation, it's advisable to consult with a healthcare professional for guidance and information tailored to their situation. Professional guidance on how to maximize your sexual life and avoid ejaculating too soon.

You just can't help but come in very quickly during sex. Just when you're at the height of passion, it ends before it's even started. Oops!

However, it's important to realize that coming rapidly is fairly normal, and most men experience premature ejaculation at some time in their lives, before writing themselves off as a sexual failure. The good news is that most guys can learn how to postpone ejaculation, and it's also readily remedied.

What is premature ejaculation?

Premature ejaculation (PE) is a common sexual dysfunction characterized by the inability to control or delay ejaculation, resulting in ejaculation occurring sooner than desired during sexual activity.

The exact time frame considered "premature" can vary, but it is generally defined as ejaculation that occurs within one minute of penetration or even before penetration in some cases.

PE can be classified into two types:

1. Lifelong PE (Primary):

This occurs from the first sexual experience and persists over time.

2. Acquired PE (Secondary):
Develops after a period of normal sexual function.

The causes of premature ejaculation can be complex and may involve psychological, biological, or interpersonal factors. It's a common condition and can affect men of all ages.

Treatment approaches may include behavioral techniques, counseling, medications, or a combination of these, depending on the underlying causes and the individual's specific situation.
If someone is concerned about premature ejaculation, seeking advice from a healthcare professional or a sex therapist is recommended.

Delayed ejaculation (DE)
Delayed ejaculation (DE), also known as male orgasmic disorder, is a condition in which a man experiences a significant delay

or inability to reach orgasm and ejaculate, despite sufficient sexual stimulation.

This delay can be distressing and may lead to frustration or dissatisfaction in sexual relationships.

Key features of delayed ejaculation include:

1. Prolonged Time:
Difficulty reaching climax, often taking an extended period of time or being unable to achieve orgasm at all.

2. Consistency:
The issue persists over an extended period and is not solely related to occasional performance anxiety.

3. Distress:
The delay causes personal distress, frustration, or difficulty in intimate relationships.

Delayed ejaculation can be caused by various factors, including psychological, physical, or relational issues.
Common contributing factors may include anxiety, depression, certain medications, hormonal imbalances, or nerve damage. Relationship issues or cultural and religious factors may also play a role.

Treatment approaches for delayed ejaculation may involve psychotherapy, behavioral therapy, medication adjustments, or addressing underlying medical conditions.
Consulting with a healthcare professional or a sex therapist is crucial for a comprehensive evaluation and personalized treatment plan.
Overcoming premature ejaculation (PE) may involve a combination of behavioral strategies, lifestyle adjustments, and, in some cases, medical interventions.

Premature ejaculation is a relatively prevalent problem in which a guy has an orgasm usually less than two minutes into the sexual encounter.
One of the most prevalent sexual anxiety disorders among men is coming too soon.
Fortunately, there are many strategies for learning to stay longer and make sure your partner is happy as well.

Most men are unaware that many guys ejaculate after just two minutes and that many more only do so for four minutes.
To maximize your sex life and extend your time in the bedroom, try using any of these strategies for having sex:

Some ways and approaches that may help to postpone Ejaculation

1. Choose a sexual posture that encourages hesitancy
Men may extend their sexual life in a variety of ways, including spooning.

Attempt to lie down beside the lady in front of you, allowing the guy to enter her from behind. Rock back and forth until you both arrive at the peak.

Because of the shallow penetration in this intimate position, it helps him last longer and prevents him from being overstimulated. It also makes you move cautiously and gently since if he gets too excited, he can lose control.

2. What is the source of your arousal from sex?

Performance anxiety may result from males worrying about their ability to have a good time in bed.

Males often feel pressure to behave a particular way, keep an erection, and take command of the situation; this may be frightening for some guys.

Consider what is causing your anxiety. It's critical to identify the specific fear you have.

It's a good idea to share your nervousness with your significant other before entering the bedroom. You might feel more intimate with each other and your nervousness can be reduced by talking things out.

3: Manage your climax by "peaking"
This is a behavioral Techniques!
-Start-Stop Technique: Practice stopping sexual stimulation for 30 seconds before resuming. Repeat as needed to delay ejaculation.
The main action in tantric sex, "peaking," is a great technique to enhance sexual performance in both sexes.
By identifying their point of no return and learning to stay just below that during sex, men can improve their control over arousal.
They then build up to the point of climax again and refrain once more. Men who frequently engage in this practice can extend their time in bed and better control their orgasm.

-Squeeze Technique: Have your partner squeeze the base of the penis for 30 seconds when you feel close to ejaculation.

It's also enjoyable to relax when you're nearly there, which intensifies the climactic orgasm.

Together, you may practice "speaking" until you both nearly reach the point of no return and then take a break.

The ideal situation would be for you to finally have a simultaneous orgasmic climax together!
Don't worry if it takes longer than expected. Enjoy your joint experimentation, since half the enjoyment is in practicing.

4. Examine orgasm retard sprays.
Premature ejaculation is momentarily relieved by desensitizing sprays and lotions. They provide a transient local numbness

that postpones ejaculation and prolongs the sexual experience.

Sprays make a great delay lubricant that helps the penis become less sensitive and last longer.

Desensitizing Products:

-Topical anaesthetics (creams or sprays) that contain lidocaine or prilocaine may help reduce sensitivity and delay ejaculation. However, they should be used cautiously and under medical guidance.

5. Use a condom to postpone having sex.

In addition to their many other advantages, condoms may postpone ejaculation by creating an additional layer of friction.

The sensation is lessened even with the thinnest condom, which allows men to last a little longer.

Please be cautious and check the condom mid-sex if you are worried that it might have ripped. Even with the best brands, the thinner the condom, the more likely it is to tear.

6. Increase masturbation to postpone erection

With premature ejaculation, masturbation may be used for or against you, so try different things to determine what works best for you.

Masturbating an hour or two before sexual activity may help delay ejaculation during intercourse.

If you take it right before a sexual encounter, you and your partner will have a longer-lasting relationship. It's likely that your next orgasm won't be quite as strong.

7. Be patient while having sex with a new person.

Many young guys are anxious about starting a relationship and don't want to seem foolish by jumping into anything too soon.

Consider whether you want to have sex with them in the first place.

If you're worried and don't feel like you can trust them to understand. Perhaps you're not at ease enough to be intimate with them if you're not at ease enough to have the conversation.

8. Practice foreplay with a feminine perspective.

Spend time making her feel good and shift the emphasis to more feminine-friendly foreplay.

Sex doesn't necessarily have to mean penetration. In any case, many women want it.

You don't have to have penetrating sex with someone to be intimate; you can focus on other forms of intimacy.

9. Play around with sex toys

Don't be scared to try new things and have fun with sex toys; they've gone a long way and offer something for everyone.

Love rings are the most popular sex toys for couples worldwide.
They are worn around the penis during lovemaking; the ring rubs against the clitoris, stimulating her more and making him last longer by limiting blood flow at the base of the penis.

You can get a decent basic silicone ring.
Vibrating love rings are very popular and provide additional stimulation during lovemaking if you want to spice things up even more.

10. Use Viagra for premature ejaculation

Although it may be helpful in the short term, Viagra shouldn't be the sole option since it isn't very practical and doesn't address the underlying problem.
Some individuals find that Viagra helps them get past their early concerns about

dating someone new; in fact, it can be just what they need to give them a push.

However, treating the underlying cause as well as the symptoms is still crucial.

11. Pelvic Floor Exercises (Kegel Exercises):

-Strengthening the pelvic floor muscles may help improve ejaculatory control. These exercises involve contracting and relaxing the muscles that support the pelvic organs.

12. Mindfulness and Relaxation Techniques:

-Learning techniques such as deep breathing, meditation, or mindfulness can help manage anxiety and stress, which are often associated with premature ejaculation.

13. Communication:

-Openly communicate with your partner about your concerns and work together to find solutions. This can reduce performance anxiety and strengthen your relationship.

14. Medical Consultation:

-If premature ejaculation persists, consulting with a healthcare professional is important. They can rule out any underlying medical conditions and discuss potential medication options.

15. Counseling or Sex Therapy:

-Professional counseling or sex therapy can address psychological factors contributing to premature ejaculation and provide coping strategies.

Remember that individual responses vary, and what works for one person may not work for another. It's advisable to seek guidance from a healthcare professional or a sex therapist to determine the most suitable approach for your specific situation.

Conclusion

My best advice is for every affected person to consult with a specialist for examination

and prescription of applicable treatments or remedies.
Preventing premature ejaculation is obtainable for sexual satisfaction in relationships.
Go for it.

Chapter Thirteen

Sexual Foreplay

Sexual foreplay refers to the activities, both physical and emotional, that occur before sexual intercourse. It involves a range of actions and interactions designed to build arousal and enhance intimacy between partners.

Foreplay is not only about physical stimulation but also about creating a connection and increasing anticipation for the main sexual act.

Any pre-intercourse sexual actions or activities are referred to as foreplay.

Common elements of sexual foreplay include:

Kissing and Caressing:
Gentle and passionate kissing, along with touching and caressing various parts of the body, helps build intimacy and arousal.

Oral Sex:
Engaging in oral sex can be a form of foreplay, providing pleasure and intensifying arousal.

Communication:
Expressing desires, fantasies, and compliments fosters emotional intimacy and can heighten the overall experience.

Erotic Massage:
Massaging and touching the body in sensual ways can enhance relaxation and arousal.

Mutual Masturbation:
Engaging in self-stimulation while in the presence of a partner can be a form of foreplay.

Role-Playing:
Exploring fantasies or taking on different roles can add excitement and anticipation to the sexual encounter.

Teasing and Playfulness:
Light teasing and playful interactions contribute to a relaxed and enjoyable atmosphere.

Foreplay is a crucial aspect of sexual activity, as it helps ensure that both partners are mentally and physically ready for the sexual experience.
It varies among individuals and couples, and communication is key to understanding and respecting each other's desires and boundaries.

Why does it matter?
For so many reasons!
The physiological and bodily reactions brought on by foreplay enable and even facilitate sexual engagement.

physiological

Although it feels nice, foreplay has deeper meanings. Foreplaying fosters an emotional connection that may strengthen your bond both inside and outside of the bedroom.

Foreplay reduces inhibitions, which might enhance the sex experience for both couples and virtual strangers.

Furthermore, some foreplay might revive your libido if stress has sapped it.

For instance, kissing causes the release of serotonin, dopamine, and oxytocin. This chemical concoction raises emotions of love, kinship, and bliss while lowering cortisol (stress hormone) levels.

Physical

By raising sexual arousal, which is different from sexual desire though it may also accomplish it, foreplay physically opens the veins.

Your body goes through many physical reactions while you are sexually aroused, such as:

- A rise in your blood pressure, pulse, and heart rate.
- Enlargement of your genitalia and other blood vessels.
- Increased blood flow to the genitalia, which results in swelling of the penis, clitoris, and labia.
- Breast enlargement and erect nipples.
- Lubricating the vagina, which may reduce discomfort and improve the pleasure of sexual activity.

First things first:

Depending on the individual, foreplay might signify various things.

Erotic stimulation before sexual intercourse is often referred to as foreplay in the context of sex.

It may even take centre stage!

You don't need much more than foreplay to get an orgasm.

Studies have long shown that a large number of vaginal donors do not have orgasm during sex alone.

Foreplay may thus be whatever you want it to be as long as the agreement is obtained.
Even better, you can begin well before things become hot.
I mean, you have to start somewhere. However, who says you have to start in the same room or even in the heat of the moment?
You may utilize foreplay to start and maintain a party if you know you'll be getting together later that day or even in a few days.
Here are a few suggestions to get you... started.

Put in a message
With a message, you may start them off without even having to be very inventive!

It should work like magic if you leave a note on their pillow or tucked away in their gym bag saying that you can't wait to get your hands filthy later.

Send a text
Texting is quick and simple, and it can be done anywhere.

Things will heat up south of the border if you send them a fast text telling them what you're going to do to them or how hot it makes you when they [fill in the gaps].

Furthermore, it conveys your thoughts to them, and who doesn't like that?

Get together for cocktails or supper.
Footsies under the table, a brief makeout session in the bathroom or parking lot, or a sly glance at what's below your clothing.

Here are a few ideas for transforming pre-party dinner or cocktails into a sexual encounter.

Play pretend

Engage in some role-playing during foreplay to turn it into an occasion to realize your most extravagant desires.

When you meet for dinner or drinks, act like you're strangers on their way to a one-night stand. Or how about acting as a mischievous nurse and doctor?

You make the decision!

Give a sincere kiss.

Don't wave them off or give them a peck of welcome. Rather, make eye contact, lean in close, and give them a long, passionate kiss.

Make sure to moan just enough to pique their interest in what's going to happen while using your hands and tongue.

Inform them that the pregame is underway.

When your goal is to strip them nude and do the most heinous act possible, there's no need to seem sly.

Express to them that you want to have them hot, hard, or wet for the day and night, using as much vivid language as possible. Schwing!

If you would want to take the lead

Desire anything more than the wham bam? With the appropriate motions, you may set the tone for foreplay or any other activity you choose.

Turn on a few candles.

Nothing sets the mood for all the sensual things quite like candles.

Tea lights are cheap, so get enough and use them in every place you could use for business.

Did we mention that candlelight looks great on the skin?

Play some tunes

Everybody has a song or two that resonates deeply with them in their unique position. Discover what theirs is, add yours for good measure, and compile other people's songs into a playlist.

Step dance

Swaying to the beat of seductive music, two bodies crushed against one another, and the sensation of each other's hot breath on your cheek. Well said.

Stripper

To do a striptease, you don't even need to have fantastic skills or a pole.

Turn down the lights and remove your garments carefully while maintaining a fearless face. It is possible to fake confidence, by the way.

Post a sensual advertisement

Arrange a picnic on the bed with a variety of delectable treats that are meant to be shared.

A dish of juicy strawberries and cherries paired with chocolate sauce and whipped cream for dipping is ideal for sharing and licking off one another.

Additionally, chocolate is naturally aphrodisiac.

Make love

Get down to business and just make out.

Try it beside the window, in the back of a taxi, or on the sofa.

It's time for the outercourse if you're already well on your way and experiencing all the good vibes.

Indeed, that does exist!

The next things you should attempt.

Massage

The body and mind may benefit much from a sensual massage since the power of touch is genuine.

Light a few candles and get out the oil, or use a dual-purpose, sometimes extremely Fifty Shades-esque massage candle.

Working your way up from their feet, be sure to touch all of their sensory pressure points and stay as long as they want.

Zones of erogenous

There are a ton of hot areas on your partner's body that are simply begging to be handled.

Go through each of their erogenous zones with a kiss, tongue, or bite.

Skin to skin

It turns out that not only lustful teenagers may enjoy dry humping.

There's nothing quite like the delicious anticipation of two bodies rubbing against one another in varying degrees of nakedness.

Express verbally

Not only does discussing your desires during intimate moments facilitate foreplay, but it also guarantees that you both get what you want and desire in bed.
Inform them of your desires and what makes you feel attracted to them.

Playthings

Sex toys are more than just big, dildo-shaped cocks.
You may use vibrators externally on every imaginable erogenous zone, regardless of their size or form.
To elevate foreplay even further, you may use finger and nipple vibrations.

Steaming shower with soap
Warm, damp flesh and palms gliding over one another's bodies as you suds up with soap?
Please say yes!
Take a hot bath as well.

Play with senses
While the tongue-twisting and monotonous humming will certainly titillate the senses, a few accessories will elevate the experience.
Put on a blindfold and tease your companion by using objects like feathers, ice cubes, and your tongue to create varying textures and temperatures.

Utilize items you already own that could feel comfortable next to your skin, or get a seduction kit.

Should you choose to go further
Are you set for your main course? Use these ideas to turn it into an absolute blast of fun.

Talking sex
Allow your lips to descend, beginning with the genitalia.
Although most of the job will be done by your lips, keep your hands active!
As you give them oral pleasure, use them to caress other areas of their body.

Heat it.
When you're in there, don't ignore the less well-known but really enjoyable parts: the frenulum, the little skin wrinkle on the bottom of the penis where the shaft meets the head, and the clitoral hood, the flap of skin covering the top of the clit.

For safe oral sex, pick up some flavored condoms and dental dams.
Delicious and responsible sex!
penetration of the vagina!
Vaginal penetration may be a stopover on the route to any other sexual act that you both like, rather than having to be the end aim.

You may use your fingers, a penis, sex toys, strap-ons, or a mix of these.

Heat it.
The penetrating partner has easy access to the receiving partner's G-spot when they execute it in a doggy style.
Additionally, the view is a plus.
Whatever is performing the penetration, lubrication is a need.
A warming lubricant will increase the penetration's heat.

Anal infiltration

If you both want to, go slow and enjoy some anal play.
Use your fingers, butt plugs, tongue, or penis to do it.
Never scrimp on lubricant!
Heat it.
It seems that being a dog is in right now!
It allows the penetrating partner easy access to the clit, penis, perineum, and prostate,

among all the other regions they would want to love at the same time.

Achieving these may also bring the receiving partner closer to experiencing an anal orgasm.

Preserve it.

Together, take a hot, soapy shower to prepare yourself fully for anal activity. Additionally, this is the ideal moment to partially open the gap with your tongue or a fingertip before closing it completely.

But what if your significant other doesn't appear to be into foreplay?

Foreplay seems to be unimportant to certain individuals.

Yes, being a slothful or self-centred partner may contribute to the issue, but it may also stem from a lack of trust in their abilities or ignorance of the ins and outs.

It's not always simple to talk about what you want in bed, particularly if you're afraid of upsetting or hurting your spouse.

Pointers to lighten the process:
Commence on a happy note.
Tell them what they're doing that makes you feel good and that you want more, instead of pointing out what they're not doing. "I love it when you kiss my neck before we have sex," as an example.
You could abuse me like that all night long.

Don't assign blame.
It will go down much better if you tell them your body is seeking something else than if you tell them they're not meeting your needs.

Demonstrate and explain.
A person sometimes needs a bit more motivation.
The next time you give them a hug or kiss, extend your embrace a little bit and let them

run their hands over your body while you tell them how wonderful it feels.

If their lack of desire for foreplay is due to ignorance, seeing a film about tantric sex together may also help push them in the right way.

Find out what people desire by asking them. Express to them how much you are turned on by them. Asking if there is anything they would want you to do more that should come up next. It's a fantastic method to start a conversation so that you may both express your desires.

Explain to them why this matters to you. It may be necessary to explain why you need foreplay and put everything out on the table.

Several things that may be pertinent to discuss are:
It makes you harder or wetter for sex.
It facilitates orgasms or makes them stronger.

Different people get aroused at different rates, and some people need longer time than others.

It brings you and them closer.

It raises awareness of pleasure zones in the body.

In summary

It's not necessary for what you see as foreplay and sex to match what you see in the media.

To enjoy, you also don't need to adhere to any schedule or sequence!

It will taste good whenever you eat it, just like dessert before supper.

Kissing is fun,

But it may also be embarrassing at times. It's crucial to get your partner's permission before doing anything and to read their body language to figure out what they like.

Everybody has to start somewhere.
Let's face it:
Kissing may be very amusing or great.
You may feel pretty awesome after a terrific kiss or make-out session, without a question.

According to science, kissing may even be beneficial to your health. Kissing has even been shown in a small 2009 research to lower perceived stress.

It is inevitable to acknowledge that not all kisses are created equal.
The concept of exchanging spit with another person may sound less than ideal if you can recall a handful of your instances.

Are you unsure about your place on the kissing spectrum?
Make sure you're ready before the big event.
Although we can't always control when the desire to kiss arises, a little planning may help a lot.

You may want to forgo the onions and garlic bread at dinner, for example, if you know that kissing is likely to occur.

Additionally, it aids in:
Verify that you don't have any cracked or dry lips. Using regular lip washes may help prevent chapped and peeling lips, particularly in the winter.
Have lip balm handy for a quick touch-up before a kiss.
To maintain a fresh taste and sensation in your mouth, chew on some gum or breath mints.
Are you concerned about your breath? Making a brief trip to the restroom to wash your teeth is perfectly acceptable.

Getty Photographs
Verify the appropriate time and location.
Though it should go without saying, it may not be the greatest idea to have a full-on makeout session on a crowded metro train.

As soon as you obtain your partner's consent—more on that later—make sure the circumstances call for a kiss.
Consider not just where but also when you want to kiss.

Did your significant other just confess they failed their last test or tell you their pet fish died? It's probably not the appropriate moment for a kiss on the forehead, but it may be consoling.
Remember to provide permission and show respect.
Although unexpected kisses in movies and TV programs may appear sweet, you should always get someone's permission before touching or kissing them.

The atmosphere may be ideal. But unless you ask, you'll never know for sure whether someone wants to kiss you or not.
It doesn't have to be uncomfortable or stiff to ask for permission, despite the common misconception that it does.

Picture the two of you, cuddling up in the corner of your preferred, darkly lit hangout, exchanging long-term lustful words.

You can't take your eyes off of them, your knees are always contacting, and you have to enlarge them to hear them speak. They abruptly stop in the middle of their question to ask, "Can I kiss you?
Their vocal tone suggests that's all they've been thinking about.
It sounds quite hot.

Some other methods to convey that you want to kiss:
Tell them, "I want to kiss you right now," while maintaining eye contact. "What are your thoughts about that?"
"I've been considering kissing you. Do you ever consider kissing me?"
Want to keep things lighthearted and informal?
In some situations, "Would you want to go out?"

Before you lean in to plant a kiss, just be sure you have a clear response.

Consent and respect go hand in hand. Accept their response politely rather than pressuring them to alter their decision or offer an explanation.

They can respond, "No," "I'd rather not," or "Maybe another time."

Inside a relationship?

You may be okay with your boyfriend kissing you out of the blue. Simply tell them it's okay to kiss you whenever they want.

When in doubt, think about the kind of kiss you want to give.

Want to express your love in public without going all out PDA?

While standing in line at the movie theatre, try giving someone a brief kiss on the shoulder.

All up for some flirting?

They may tremble if there is a trail of kisses left on their neck.

Recall that it's not necessary to kiss someone on the lips each time.

Rather than coming on hard right away, it's generally preferable to start slowly and develop tension.

You're prepared to take action after you've mastered the fundamentals. ·

It doesn't have to be difficult to kiss.

As usual, begin with the fundamentals if you're anxious about doing it correctly.

Ask questions always

Make sure you're interpreting the scenario right before planting your first kiss by asking out loud.

From there, you have the option of using both words and actions to establish the tone or using your body language to go closer or cup their cheek.

Not only is consent crucial.

It may also be quite seductive.

Pull in,

Do you feel a bit uneasy?

Take your time, particularly if you are unsure of how to angle your head.

If you're concerned about your partners' foreheads colliding, softly tilt your head or move their face to the side.
Although it's not necessary to stare them down, maintaining eye contact for a few moments might help the first move seem less uncomfortable.

Take it easy.
Simply begin the kiss by using soft, gradual, and delicate pressure.

Would you want to keep kissing?
Try slowly changing the pressure to lengthen and build it up.
Moreover, you may change your attention from their upper lip to their lower lip.
Recall that little pressure always goes a long way.

Maintain a relaxed mouth.
Try not to kiss too firmly or force a pucker.

When in doubt, mimic your partner's actions since most individuals like their kisses.
Imagine a nice kiss as a conversation between two people, not just one.

Make use of your hands
At first, hand placement may seem a bit strange, but go with what is most comfortable for you.
Attempt putting your hands over your partner's neck, stroking their hair with one, or going to each location with one hand.

You may always place your hands on your partner's hips or lower back if there's a height difference but don't think too hard about it.

If you'd want to switch up your kissing style from closed to open-mouth

When you're ready to step it up a notch or two, these pointers will make the switch from closed-mouth to open-mouth kissing very effortless.

Begin at the tongue's tip.
When it comes to everything tongue-related. The majority of individuals dislike having saliva on their faces.
Try putting your tongue tip against theirs for quick, gentle contact.
Don't even attempt to stick your whole tongue in their mouth.
There's more to an unexpected tongue in your mouth than simply a mouthful of saliva. It's also really unattractive, and you may be bitten sometimes.

Discover your natural rhythm.
Naturally, remember to breathe, and discover what feels comfortable for you and your partner. Uncertain about whether they want to continue or take a break?
Asking never hurts.

If you want an intense make-out session,
Depending on the circumstance, sharing a kiss might quickly become rather passionate. Go ahead and do more if you and your partner feel comfortable doing so!
Be mindful of your body language.
Physical indications like drawing away or getting closer might reveal more about your partner's preferences.
Not everyone utilizes nonverbal signs, particularly when their mouth is busy. That implies that by closely observing your spouse, you may find out more about what is (and isn't) working.

Don't lead the kissing party to an exclusive advantage for yourself.
A kiss that brings happiness to both parties is the nicest kind.

Increase the intensity gradually.
It's not necessary to go headfirst into a passionate make-out session. However, you

may not want to hold onto a single kiss for
too long.

Develop the kiss gradually into something
more.
Don't be scared to communicate your
preferences to your spouse via body
language.
Nonverbal communication is crucial as well.
Maintain eye contact before, during, and
after kissing.
Although it's rather customary to kiss with
your eyes closed, you don't have to do so the
whole time.

It's okay to glance at your spouse in between
kisses. It's best to avoid making strong eye
contact during a kiss unless you are certain
that your spouse loves it.
Away from their lips for a moment.
Change places without fear as the kiss
intensifies.
A satisfying kiss might consist of many
kisses on the earlobe, collarbone, or jawline.

Be careful if you decide to bite someone.

It's normally better to keep to a moderate pull on the lips since not everyone feels comfortable biting their lips during a kiss. Anything beyond that may be worth discussing to see what both of you are comfortable with.

To intensify the situation even more

It's always a good idea to discuss various types of intimacy and what you wish to create with your partner, even if you're just enjoying the act of kissing as part of foreplay.

Oral or penetrative intercourse does not have to result from every kiss. It's OK for a kiss to sometimes simply be a kiss.

Move in closer if you haven't already.

Remove any gap between you and your companion whenever you're ready to intensify your kiss.

However, keep in mind that while being physically close to someone might feel amazing, mental closeness can strengthen your bond.

Examine other erogenous zones

Although there are many "feel-good" spots on the body, not everyone will find them in the same areas.

Learn about your partner's many erogenous zones, such as their neck or ears. Observe their responses to see which areas they are most receptive and sensitive to.

If you want to progressively work your way up to anything bigger, you may even move to various sections of the body.

Increase the amount of time you spend utilizing your hands.

Sharing a kiss may indeed be a full-body sensation.

Therefore, don't be scared to caress your partner's arms or back, run your hands through their hair, or hug them close.

Regardless of the kiss, feedback is essential. A crucial component of every kiss is communication. It facilitates mutual understanding between you and your spouse, allowing you to enjoy kissing in a manner that makes everyone happy.

While you may provide or receive feedback orally or nonverbally during a kiss, you can also subtly communicate later by stating things like:

I enjoyed it when you did.

[Blank] had a great feeling.

We ought to attempt more or less of this the next time.

Did you like my attempt at it?

Is it OK if we...

I don't know whether I feel at ease around. Should we try reducing that?

You may want to tell someone how much you enjoyed yourself but are at a loss for words. Never forget that there are always other ways to express your love for your spouse, including holding their hand, petting their hair, or giving them a strong embrace.

Express your love in many ways.
Perhaps after a passionate make-out session, your lips have gone numb, or your partner wants to postpone the kiss.
It never hurts to express your interest and care in less tangible ways, regardless of the situation.

Suggestions to consider:
Give a sincere compliment. "I like being in your company."
"I constantly laugh with you", and "I enjoy our time together so much."
Use words to convey your desire for a kiss. Not exactly the proper moment or location for a kiss?
Create anticipation by noting in a message that you are eager to kiss them later, or by telling them as much.

Together, go for a stroll. You might offer to keep them company if they're leaving for a snack, their house, or the office.

Look for a spot to put your head down. Perhaps you want to continue caressing, but you also want to focus on the film.

If you're taller and you want to stay in touch without being completely preoccupied, you may lean your head on their head or shoulder, depending on how tall you are.

Join hands.

When you're ready to go on to kissing, hand holding could feel a bit too subdued, but remember your very first handshake. Recall the sensation of your fingers brushing against one other, or the chill you felt as they ran their finger over your hand?

Your hands may also convey a great deal about how you are feeling.

In summary

There are several reasons why we kiss, but mostly because it may feel so good.

Consequently, you would certainly agree that the finest kisses are those that you and your spouse love sharing.

Remember that these are just recommendations.
You are free to use as many or as few of them as desired.
The key to enjoying a fantastic kiss is communication with your partner; otherwise, there's no right or wrong way to do it.

Chapter Fourteen

The Foreplay That Women Loves

Similar to exercising, having sex may be unpleasant and even hazardous if neither partner has fully warmed up for the other. Although we understand how eager you are to get to the juicy parts, foreplay has its benefits as well. You will come to love the pre-game just as much as the big finish if you put in the necessary time and effort.
Actual women get excited in foreplay motions and the males should learn corresponding motions to make foreplay inventive and engaging.

After speaking with actual women about what motivates them, they have these to say about foreplay

1. Speak with me
I'm all for a guy who can talk during foreplay.

While moaning and groaning are OK, having a humorous conversation about dirty work may be enjoyable for both of you and usually results in obtaining more or less of what you need in the bedroom.

It's a fantastic way to energize me.

2. Keep an eye on the twins

When they don't give their breasts adequate attention, it stinks.

The majority of men seem to be content to spend a considerable amount of time in various foreplay situations and activities, but they essentially simply glance at the boobs, give them a cursory glance, and then walk on, seldom coming back.

It is rather depressing.

Give them extra affection; it's nice!

3. Show kindness

Some simply jump right in and attempt to click on my clitoral area like it's a computer mouse before I've even taken off my clothes.

I thought I was hooking up with Jack the

Ripper when one man got very rowdy with his fingers.

Guys, unwind—this is a turn-on.

4. Take Off My Clothing

In and of itself, undressing someone is a kind of foreplay.

It seems like the sexiest element of having an intimate relationship.

It is, of course, a bit upsetting when a man becomes so enthused about the outcome that I end up removing my clothing too quickly.

5. Reinstall the tongue in your mouth

While the tongue may be highly seductive and entertaining, using it excessively might be harmful.

This also applies to tongue involvement in all bodily regions.

Mouth (kisses should incorporate the tongue as well as the lips, not just the tongue), ears (though this can also be sultry, it could go wrong and give me the impression that you're cleaning my ears with your tongue), neck (neck kisses are lovely, but please don't slobber all over me like a dog or leave hickeys after middle school—I have to go to work with that), and finally, lady parts (extremely important—tongue is crucial but needs to be utilized correctly).

6. Give It Your All
No one will benefit from the sex if I am not fully warmed up.
It may even cause pain.
Enjoy the delight of being goofy, and just be present in the moment.
The good stuff is on the way (pun intended).

7. Make Use of Both Hands
Thus, you have another free hand, even if you are using one down there.
Go for my breasts, my posterior, or even simply give me a little touch in any way.
Avoid becoming indolent.

8. Multiple Tasking

There's nothing more uncomfortable than a man gazing at me and fingering me at the same time.

Kiss me!

Where it is, I could care less, but don't simply creepily lay there.

Why is juggling those two tasks at the same time so difficult?

9. Savor My Morning Ritual

It's for you if I'm wearing anything frilly.

If you can't tell, I squandered a whole day in an uncomfortable bra and perfectly nice underpants.

Please don't hurry things so much that you overlook how attractive I am in my underwear.

You may not have the chance to see it again, so take a moment to appreciate everything.

10. A Small Bite

Here, "nibble" is crucial.

Under no circumstances should you handle my skin like jerky steak.
However, it's very hot when someone lightly bites my neck, lip, nipple, or ear.
That being said, my downstairs area is not covered by this.

Chapter Fifteen

Body Areas That You Must Never Ignore When Engaging in Foreplay

You will want to visit these wonderful locales, I promise.

Friends, it's about time we quit using foreplay as a means to sleep.

It has the power to transform a "good" sexual encounter into a mind-blowing, fully immersive, almost religious one.

Indeed, it is that significant.

You'll be set up for better sex from head to toe if you slow down and prioritize all the nice things that far too many of us try to hurry right over on the way to downtown. Engaging in foreplay not only helps to increase desire by increasing blood flow to the genitalia but also helps to clear your thoughts and prepare you for amazing sex.

Not to confuse us, but I also need to completely abandon the phrase "foreplay" for now.

It puts penetrating sex at the pinnacle of a sexual hierarchy, that isn't very helpful for getting the greatest enjoyment out of it sex.

In case you missed it, external clitoral stimulation causes orgasms in the great majority of individuals with clitorises.

Sure, penis in vegina is entertaining, but it's not everything.

As long as everyone is having fun, then all sexual activity is equal.

Anything outside of penetration should truly be referred to as "moreplay."

This implies that there is more to genuinely fantastic, toe-curling sex than just genitalia. Exploring the vast range of erogenous zones opens up a plethora of opportunities for experiencing pleasure.

An erogenous zone is an area where you feel sexually or erotically awakened when touched, stroked, kissed, bit, or sucked.

Consider your inner arms, neck, foot, lower back, and other areas.

Everyone has a varied preference for where and how they want to be touched; therefore, there is no right or wrong method to explore these various body parts.

Are you unsure about where to start your exploratory journey?

You are in good hands here!

To enhance your foreplay experiences and elevate your sexual interactions, try these locations and body regions.

1. The vicinity of the eyes

The region around your penis may be just as sensuous and sexual as the typical portions of your body that are most often sexualized as erogenous zones.

Lightly stroke their eyebrows with your thumbs and plant tender kisses on their eyelids.

This kind of gentle face-stroking and deep eye contact can lead to a great deal of intimacy.

2. Area of the inside bicep and tricep

This area is not only very sexual and sensitive, but it's also a simple pleasure place to stimulate.

Softly massage the region by making circular movements with your tongue.

Use that area to drive your partner crazy because the skin there gets thinner.

It feels better when less pressured.

3. The collarbone

The clavicle and the grooves below it can be highly responsive to light touch.

Even though it's an inconspicuous area of your body, your partner may utilize it to arouse you in ways you were unaware of.

Run the backs of your fingers over the bone and run your tongue along the underside of them.

4. The toes

To be honest, before you start shrimpin', you should ask your partner whether they're OK with any foot or toe play.

Whether or not you end up being kicked in the face. However, licking or sucking them can be extremely erotic because toes are very sensitive.

5. The lobes of the ears

Many individuals have very sensitive ears and earlobes.

A major turn-on can be giving someone sexy talk, nibbling on their earlobes, licking behind their ear, or blowing gently in their ear, certain assigned female at birth people may even have eargasms from this kind of stimulation alone.

6. The canal of the inner ear

Though it may seem strange.

The inner ear may feel quite wonderful and be very sensitive.

Have you ever cleaned your ears and experienced that amazing, almost sensual feeling?

Yes, it's about safely investigating that feeling.

Touch this region in a manner that is more sensuous than just putting your finger in there to glob out some earwax.

To release a body tingling sensation that will have your partner moaning, glide your finger in slowly and give it a little twist or even a light shake back and forth, little nibbling of the earlobe may complement this kind of stimulation quite nicely.

You don't want to create pain or suffering, so take it very gently. It is detrimental to your ears to get to the rear of the canal. Proceed with care!

7. In the back of the knees

When massaged or stroked softly, the sensitive region behind the knee may respond quite well.

Making eye contact with your partner may intensify the intoxicating effects of this, experiment with this by using different kinds of strokes with the fingertips or the entire finger.
Your spouse might go crazy over it!

Remember that some individuals may find this region quite sensitive, or even ticklish, so make sure you consult your spouse before spending a lot of time touching the backs of their knees. Often, we may change our experience of touch from an unpleasant one to a sensuous one by being conscious of what we're about to do instead of simply going for it blindly.
We like seeing consent!

8. The hair

The scalp contains a lot of nerve endings; therefore, it should be on your list of sensitive spots.
Who doesn't like a nice head massage, after all?

Softly grasping their hair at the nape of their neck or running your hands through their hair.

If your significant other enjoys pulling hair, you may also experiment with that.
Try pulling and tugging your partner's hair; start gently and see how hard they like it.
As with any sex experiment, be sure to follow up to make sure your partner is having fun.

9. Shoulders and back of the neck

The back of the neck and shoulders are reached by moving down from the scalp to the nape of the neck.
This region may appear to be very sensitive to gentle tickling.
Arousal may also be increased with some mild nibbles or love bites if you and your partner are game lovers.

10. Hands

Another crucial body component to concentrate on during foreplay is your hands.

We have the same number of nerve endings in our hands as in our genitalia.

Close your partner's eyes, take their hands, and gently lead them to wipe their fingers over your face, down over your neck, shoulders, breasts, and any other sensitive areas.

Tell them precisely how you want to be touched by using touch.

11. The rectum

A genuinely pleasurable tantric massage begins with stimulating your partner's surrounding body before focusing on their genitalia and causing them to climax,

A tantric massage, a little massage of the pubic bone may release a wealth of sensual potential.

When you're ready to work on more intense erogenous zone stimulation, you may start

by using a few fingers to gently massage the perineum, which is the region between the penis and the butthole.
Try this one baby while keeping his penis pressed up against his body.

12. The heel
While working on the public bone, you may also focus on extra erogenous zone stimulation by using a couple of fingers to gently massage the perineum, which is the region between the penis/vulva and anus.
Try this one while holding your partner's penis up against their body.
This will surely get the juices flowing.
If your spouse has a vulva, you may use your fingers to touch the external clitoris while softly massaging the perineum with your knuckles in a rocking motion.

13. The very delicate lip-border
There is untapped potential for the buccal nerve, which surrounds the mouth's margins, to get stimulated during a kiss.

This area is extremely sensitive to touch, but it's often overlooked since most people focus on the plump part of the lips.

You'll feel tingling, almost ticklish, if you attempt delicately tracing the tip of your finger around the corners of your lips (like you're applying lip liner).

You may enjoy the pleasures of making out without having to lick your partner's whole mouth—that would be awkward. Rather, kiss as usual and then delicately trace the edge of the top lip with the tip of your tongue.

Drawback and give them another playful kiss, then trace the outline of their lower lip.

14. The nipples

Nipple play has benefits, this zone may be particularly enjoyable to explore since the nipples are often "uncharted territory—an erogenous zone we haven't really experimented with."

Nipple play may be really enjoyable for assigned female at birth people since it can be a very sensitive spot to touch.

Some people may truly have an orgasm just by playing with their nipples since it activates the same part of the brain as vaginal stimulation—the genital cortex.
The connection may be so deep for some who get nipple gas that they can build up enough sexual tension in their bodies to experience that exquisite release.

Additionally, by playing it out with your partner, you may express to them precisely what you want done to your body.
Whatever makes those nips pop may be used to gently flick them with your tongue, bite them, or rub them.
Never forget to stop by and make sure everyone is enjoying themselves.

15. The sensual dip where the neck and chest meet

There's an erogenous zone stretching from your jawline to your shoulders, but one spot in particular will give you more goosebumps than the rest.

 It's that little indentation where the neck connects with the collarbone.
The sensations are stronger there because the skin is thinner and there is less fatty tissue underneath, it feels very pleasant to touch this place.

Follow the tips of your index and middle fingers from one shoulder to the dip in the middle as you kiss down their neck.
Take your time and slowly, circularly move your fingers. Then, as you warm the area with your breath, glide your tongue over the location and plant a kiss.

16. The torso's sides

A strong nerve that runs from the base of the rib cage to the hips is directly connected to your clitoris and the penis or vulva of your partner when it is activated.

In people of all genders, this part of the body reflexively causes the pelvic floor muscles to contract, which increases arousal.

This area is more sensitive than other places; therefore, you should apply extra pressure there.

Beginning on the side just under the rib cage, move your hand in a stroking motion or alternate between softly nibbling and kissing (pressing down harder than normal) your way down to the hip bone.

17. The heap on the backside

Due to its abundance of nerves, the base of the spine's knob has a high arousal potential. Give each other a massage to benefit from each other.

Knead with your hands starting at the shoulder blades and working your way down.
Use a gentler touch and gently spiral your fingers around the base at the lower back.
Since this region is so sensitive, even the slightest contact may cause shivers to go down your body.

You may also delicately dab your face against the region; the unexpected contact of skin on the skin causes dopamine, the hormone associated with excitement, to rise.
Next, place a little kiss there and move your tongue over the same area.
To intensify the feeling, try brushing the tips of your hair against the skin. After that, try lightly scraping your fingernails over it.

18. The groove on the lower legs
At the top of the inner thigh sits one of the body's most explosive nerves.

It's known as the ilioinguinal nerve, and it's extremely sensitive to touch.

It's preferable to reserve it for last and ascend to it gradually.
To begin, lick your finger (the moisture intensifies the pleasure) and move it gently up your leg from the mid-inner to the top. Then, using your tongue to guide you, follow the line you have drawn to the top area.

Chapter Sixteen

Foreplay Tricks for Men

Men and women like foreplay equally.

It's fantastic.

Continue having fun for as long as you both feel like it.

It is crucial to fully warm up before engaging in any physically demanding activity.

So why not make the most of your pre-intercourse enjoyment while you can? There are a lot of sultry elements that will enhance the next release.

When actual males where asked about what motivates them sexually, check out the results:

1: Show Him Some Strips

She makes sure I see her undressed whenever she wants me to remember how hot she is.

She lifts her skirt over her thighs and takes off her stockings, pulling them down with

her hands sliding up her calves. She then began to carefully undo her blouse, flashing me seductive glances in between each button.
At last, the straps come off her shoulders as she undoes her bra and cups her breasts.
It drives me crazy.

2: Put on your Grove
She grabs me, puts the stereo on full blast, and starts dancing around the house with me.
It's so romantic; there's something so seductive about it.

3: Put your cow or cat ahead.
I like her stretching and subsequent all-fours poses.

4: Utilize a Toy

I enjoy seeing my baby playing with her vibrator when I enter my bedroom.

5: Sends sexy text
Now and then she would text me and say, 'I want to [bleep] tonight.'
I like receiving witty, sinister letters like this one.
It assures me that she will be prepared to go when I get home.

6: Give Him a Gift Card as a Surprise
She recently gave me a Victoria's Secret gift card.
"Let's go shopping; you can buy anything you want me to wear,"
Having the last say over the purchases we made was a fantastic perk.

7: Engage in footsie.
My spouse is an expert player of footsie.
She often sports high heels, and she likes to rub her foot along my calf, first on the outside and then the inside of my leg.

Then she takes off her shoes and uses her bare feet to caress my legs.

My ankles tingle from her toes.

She places her bare feet on my lap whether we're at home or in the dimly lit rear booth of our favorite local bar, and I find it difficult to get back up for a while.

8: Include a Calendar Event

One day, after working long hours, I opened my work date planner and saw a note written on the page for that day that wrote, 'Sex @ 7pm' One night, she must have pulled my calendar out of my briefcase and scrawled something in it. Needless to say, I arrived home promptly that evening.

9: Continue wearing your coat

My wife refused to take off her coat one evening when we were out to supper and seated at a table.

She replied that she couldn't when I asked why, and then she simply looked at me.

It turned out that her only clothing choices were high heels and a trench coat.

This is the sexiest thing I've ever seen, that was all I could think about as I was unable to even eat.

10: Kiss Him to Get His Attention

She once placed her head on my lap as we were watching a movie, grabbed my hand, and kissed each of my fingers softly while maintaining eye contact.

I stopped the movie since it was obvious what was on her mind.

11: Proceed in This Direction

She walks in a unique style that's reserved only for me; she strolls about gently, her hips undulating in different directions.

She wears her high heels for ten or fifteen minutes after she gets home from work, just long enough for her to know that I'm noticing her attractive stroll.

I want to show her to the bedroom right now.

12: Engage in the Whisper Game.

My wife may sometimes whisper sweet words in my ear, such as, 'you look sexy in that clothing,' or 'I love you.'

Then she delicately places my earlobe between her teeth and flicks the inside of my ear with the tip of her tongue.

Every time, it makes me shiver down my spine.

13: Put Some Friction in It

With my wife on my arm, I felt confident at the black-tie event we were attending at a museum.

She gently nuzzled one of her breasts on my arm as we studied an artwork.

She repeated the action in the next picture, then again in front of the sculpture.

We were both trying not to laugh at this point since the affluent audience had no idea that we were being sly, which made her subtle seduction even more alluring.

After sharing a brief kiss in an empty art space, we made the quickest trip to get our outerwear.

14: Employ a Nanny

My wife sometimes surprises me with the nicest kind of gift: an at-home sex date. "I'll know precisely what our plans are for that evening," she'll murmur. "The kids are sleeping at the babysitter's overnight."

15: Extract the Razor

She enjoys shaving my facial hair before we have sex.

Having her body so close to mine as she runs the razor over my face is sensuous and personal.

It's also very nurturing; we usually end up slobbering over one another afterward.

16: Advise him to take a nap.

She groaned loudly, got up from the sofa, and said she was going to take a nap.
She turned to face me over her shoulder as she went away, obligingly taking off her clothing.
She was nude on the bed when I arrived in the bedroom.
I started to kiss her while she kept on "sleeping." It's like a sexual dream come true."

17: Give Him a Drink

She'll pour us each a Scotch on the rocks and light candles in the bedroom.
After that, we chat while drinking in bed before making love.
I felt extremely Cary Grant-like after this event.

18: Act as if you are a stranger.

She started playing a little game with me while we were out to supper. She started asking me questions and making out with me like we were on a blind date.

I thought this was ridiculous at first, but I went along with it.

She shed all of her inhibitions in a matter of minutes, telling me the "stranger" things she had never uttered to me before and even describing her favorite parts of having sex.

I was quite thrilled.

Playing along with her in this manner reminded me of the excitement of the pursuit and made me realize how much I wanted to take our "date" to bed.

That evening, we had the craziest sex.

19: Make a Small Lip Motion

I adore her hand-kissing technique.

She holds it first and runs a thumb over its back.

She then brings my hand to her lips, pressing them first on my palm and then the back of it. Then, as if she were taking my pulse with her lips, she pressed her mouth to the inside of my wrist.

It consistently raises the heart rate.

20: Make a Trace After You

My wife contacted me one evening when I was in the living room.

I saw an arrow pointing toward the bed at the end of a string of Hershey's Kisses that led to the master bedroom as I was walking down the hallway.

She wanted to do more for me that evening than simply kiss me.

Chapter Seventeen

Introduction To Sexuality

For various individuals, sex may signify different things.

Having intercourse should be enjoyable for all parties involved; it's not only about becoming pregnant.

Ensuring everyone wants to participate, feels protected, and enjoys the activity throughout, is what it means to provide consent.

Knowing each other's anatomy will make it easier for you to enjoy yourself during sex.

STIs are widespread and not a cause for shame. Every STI has a treatment. Many are treatable.

Without sex, we wouldn't be here on Earth. Even though it's a natural part of life, many individuals still believe it inappropriate to talk about sex. Many questions and confusion may arise from this.

Finding what suits you and what your tastes are takes time. It's OK!

Since we are all on unique timelines, no two people's paths to sexual pleasure are the same.

Do you want to have sex but don't know where to begin?

The bare minimum that you should be aware of is provided here.

What is sexual activity?

Any action that involves one, two, or more persons and makes them feel aroused (sexually stimulated) is called sex.

It may be verbal, tactile, or both.

It doesn't always need touching genitalia, although it may.

When individuals discuss sex, they often refer to penetrating sex or sexual encounters.

Every participant in a sexual activity should find it delightful, and permission should be given at all times.

Facts about consenting to sex

You may not even be aware of sexual consent, even if you have heard of it.

This implies that, at the start of the activity, everyone should decide what they are comfortable with.

It is crucial that someone be allowed to express a change of heart or decide they want to quit, and that their decision is accepted.

This guarantees that everyone's experience will be enjoyable.

Which kinds of sex?

1. Sexual activity via the vagina

When the penis touches, penetrates, or rubs against another vagina, it is known as vaginal intercourse.

2. oral to vaginal sex

Also known as "oral sex." The genitalia are stimulated or made pleasurable by the tongue.
You may do this by sucking, kissing, or licking.

3. Anal intercourse

The anus (butthole) is where the penis or sex toy is placed.
Because the anus cannot produce its own lubricant, lubrication is crucial.

4. Erogenous contact

It is possible to elicit a sexual emotion or experience using the hands or other body parts. This may include touching and massaging the genitalia or other regions of the body, as well as nipple stimulation, kissing, and snuggling.

5. Handjobs or fingering

Fingering is the act of stimulating the clitoris, inserting the fingers into the vagina or the anus, or any combination of these, to elicit sexual sensations.

Using a hand to stimulate the penis is known as a hand job.

6. Masturbation

Groping for sex by touching your body parts. You may work on this by yourself or in tandem with another person.

A variety of sex toys, such as vibrators, dildos, anal toys, and more, may be used during masturbation.

7. Video/phone sex

Engaging in sexually stimulating conversation, flirtation, and picture exchange over the phone or the internet.

What is sex desire and where does it originate?

The urge to have sex is known as libido, or sex drive.

Our sexual desire is influenced by hormones, stress levels, and our physical and emotional well-being.

Our thoughts about sex and pleasure might change throughout our lives due to the impact of our sexual partners, family, friends, community, and faith or religion.

Orgasm and sexual pleasure

There is no one definition of sexual pleasure.

Numerous things might make you happy and satisfied.

An extreme ecstasy is known as an orgasm. Here's one method for getting good sex:

When the penis hardens and enlarges, those with penises have orgasms. This happens when the body releases hormones in response to a desire for sexual activity. Usually, ejaculation happens during an orgasm.

When the clitoris (and sometimes the inner and outer labia) are aroused and swell, people with vulvas have orgasms.

The clitoris contains a high concentration of nerve endings, much like the penis.

The body sends messages to the nerves by touching and rubbing these erogenous zones.

Feelings of pleasure may be sent throughout the body via this.

It's critical to comprehend the anatomy of both you and your partner to maximize your enjoyment during sex.

Additionally, communication is essential. Something comfortable for you may not be for someone else.

Discuss your likes and dislikes with your spouse.

Experimenting to determine the most pleasurable touches may be entertaining. Intimacy may rise along with more communication.

Another method that could assist you in understanding the optimal approaches to sexual satisfaction is masturbation.

How to engage in safer sexual activity
You can lower your risk of STIs and pregnancy by having safer sex.
The primary kind of sexual activity that may result in pregnancy is penis-in-vagina.
In addition, if semen enters the vagina during another kind of sexual activity, pregnancy may result.
During all types of intercourse, when bodies and bodily fluids come into contact, STIs may be transferred.

The best defenses against STIs (Sexually Transmitted Illnesses) are as follows:

1. Every time you have sex, use barrier techniques correctly. The use of barrier techniques on toys and body parts is advised for any oral, anal, or vaginal intercourse.

Among the barrier techniques are:

External condoms, sometimes referred to as "male" condoms,

Condoms inside (sometimes referred to as "female" condoms)

Nitrile or latex gloves

dental dams

2. Make liberal use of condom-safe lubricant

3. Before alternating between anal, vaginal, or oral intercourse, change condoms.

4. When exchanging sex toys, use sterile or fresh condoms.

5. Regularly check for any STIs, and urge your partner to do the same

The risk of contracting an STI is greatly reduced by barrier techniques.
They function by keeping the genitalia and bodily fluids of each partner away from the body of the other.
Condoms may also prevent conception around 98% of the time with perfect usage and 87% of the time with normal use when used consistently.

Unless both partners have recently tested negative for an STI and you are both positive and have not had intercourse with anyone else since the test, you should always utilize a barrier technique.
Use a condom each time you have sex if you want to avoid becoming pregnant.

No glove, no love: condom haggling and popular justifications

Condoms are a highly useful tool for avoiding sexually transmitted infections and pregnancy.

What happens if my spouse refuses to wear a condom?

It's important to safeguard your health and enjoy all aspects of sexual activity. Communicate honestly and openly with your spouse.

Consider if you want to remain with them if they push you to have risky sexual relations.

Symptoms,
Treatment options, and
Prevention of STIs and STDs

The experience of having an STI

STIs are a frequent and diverse occurrence. We made contact via social media.

Over a million sexually transmitted infections (STIs) are acquired globally each day.

STIs are quite widespread, but how much do you know about them?

Were you aware that there are precautions you may take to avoid getting STIs?

Did you know that a lot of sexually transmitted infections have little or no symptoms?

You can modify the safety measures you use regarding sex in your own life if you are aware of some simple facts.

Chlamydia
Since chlamydia often has no symptoms, many individuals are unaware that they have it.

The symptoms of chlamydia might include yellow discharge that resembles pus, painful or frequent urination, spotting during or after intercourse, and/or discomfort, bleeding, or discharge from the rectal area.

If left untreated, it may cause ectopic pregnancy, persistent pelvic discomfort, pelvic inflammatory illness, and/or infertility in females and those with female reproductive tracts.

Herpes genital

The second-most prevalent STI in the United States is genital herpes.

Certain individuals with herpes get repeated blisters and ulcers in their vaginal regions.
Many herpes patients don't exhibit any symptoms, allowing them to go on transmitting the infection.
Herpes has no known cure, yet outbreaks and symptoms may be controlled.

Gonorrhea

Since gonorrhoea often has no symptoms, many individuals are unaware that they have it.

If left untreated, it may cause ectopic pregnancy, persistent pelvic discomfort, pelvic inflammatory illness, and/or infertility in females and those with female reproductive tracts.

The trichomonas infection
Since trichomoniasis often has no symptoms, many individuals are unaware that they have it.

How does vaginal discharge vary throughout the cycle, and what does it mean?

Cervical fluid types vary in terms of quality, consistency, and volume in tandem with...

Increased, malodorous, colorful vaginal discharge, vulvar soreness and itching, and/or pain during urination or sexual activity are among the symptoms that some individuals may encounter.

HIV
HIV may spread via the sharing of certain body fluids, such as vaginal fluids, breast milk, semen, and blood.

HIV cannot be spread by sneezing, crying, saliva, or direct touch.

HIV may be spread via unprotected anal, penis-in-vagina, and sometimes even oral intercourse.

HIV cannot be cured, although there are drugs that can maintain a low viral load and significantly lower the risk of HIV infection and transmission.

Which sexual behaviors may spread sexually transmitted infections?

Semen, vaginal secretions, skin-to-skin contact, blood, saliva, and even excrement may all spread STIs.

People commonly participate in many forms of sexual activity (e.g., oral sex and penis-in-vagina intercourse in the same session), making it difficult to determine which sex act is responsible for the spread of illness.

STIs acquired by kissing

Herpes oral (HSV-1)

Oral sex might expose you to STIs.

chlamydia

gonorrhoea

HPV

HSV-1 and HSV-2 herpes

Syphilis

HIV

The trichomonas infection

STIs that may result from anal and vaginal fisting and fingering

Blood-borne STIs (such as HIV or hepatitis B or C) are more likely to spread if anything may cut or rip the skin around the anus or genitals, such as fingernails, rings, or skin ripping.

STIs may spread via genital fluids if your fingers come into contact with someone else's genitalia before touching your own. Always wash your hands after handling someone else's genitalia to ensure safety, and you may also use gloves for further protection.

STIs may be contracted during vulva-to-vulva or penis-in-vaginal intercourse.

HIV

gonorrhoea

chlamydia

HSV-1 and HSV-2 herpes

HPV

Syphilis

Chancroid

Hepatitis B and C

The trichomonas infection

Warts on the genitalia

STIs that arise from anal intercourse

HIV

Hepatitis B and C

HPV

Syphilis

gonorrhoea

chlamydia

HSV-1 and HSV-2 herpes

Warts on the genitalia

illnesses spread by bacteria found in faeces, including Giardia, Shigella, Salmonella, Campylobacter, and E. coli

A STI is not something to be embarrassed about.

In addition to being vital for your sexual health, talking openly about STIs with peers and informing your partners may help combat stigma and shatter taboos associated with society and culture.
Choosing when and how to have sex is up to you.
Your sexual encounters may be enjoyable and exciting if you are secure, comfortable, and knowledgeable.

Chapter Eighteen

A Comprehensive Guide To Having Sexual Intercourse

Are you going to have sex?

Here's a step-by-step breakdown of the full performance.

Even though having sex may be fulfilling and enjoyable, there are a few things to consider if you're planning to do it for the first time and are unsure of where to begin. Here's a step-by-step instruction on how to have sex to help you crack that sexual code.

Step 1:
Determine if the individual desires sex too:

The most crucial element of a satisfying sexual encounter is this.

The whole procedure may go south if one of the couples is not feeling sexually inclined or wants to have sex.

Not to mention that it may give you or your partner a feeling of being taken advantage of or violated.

Decide whether or not they want to have sex.

A few frequent signs to watch out for include if the individual appears eager to touch you, gets closer to you, or seems enthusiastic about being with you physically.

Even while they are indicators, keep in mind that you shouldn't misinterpret them and that sometimes the best way to find out is to ask.

Step 2:
Get ready:
It's fantastic having sex. It is enjoyable and brings you joy.

It also helps you burn calories and overcome sadness, among many other health advantages.

It makes sense that humans are the only species whose sexual activity is done for enjoyment rather than just reproduction. However, issues like unintended pregnancies, STDs, and emotional disappointments accompany all of that enjoyment.

So your best bet is to be ready.

Have the contraceptive pill, carry a condom, and keep in mind that you must be psychologically prepared for the act.

People become closer over sex.

That is just the nature of human biology.

So keep in mind that you should have your head in alignment with your body's desires whether you are taking the first step towards a serious relationship or arranging a one-night stand.

Talking about it is a wonderful method to do this.

Talk to your partner about what you think this could lead to, ask them if they have protection (if not, go buy some, there are plenty of options available), and most importantly, be honest about how you view the act (i.e., whether it's something you want to do for fun with no commitments or something more serious). Recall that condoms are intended to be used just once. Make sure you get extra condoms in case you want to use them more than once since you cannot use one twice.

Step 3:
Decide on the setting and create the atmosphere:

Sexual activity is, or should be, a private matter.

Choose a location where you can both be yourselves, particularly if this is the first time.

Select a quiet location with a cozy area for sexual activity.

Having a cozy, well-made bed and mood lighting is usually beneficial (unless you want to take risks).

Thus, indulge a little.

Recall that enjoyment has a price.

Step 4:
Don't come off as very desperate and approach the individual gently:

One of the greatest turn-offs is coming on too hard or being pushy about getting into a relationship.

Therefore, even if you are yearning to be with someone, avoid coming off as desperate and give them room to express their emotions.

It's important to express your desire for physical intimacy, but if you don't believe the other person is interested, back off.

Let them make their own decisions about sex.

You might just ask them if you are near enough to them.

It will be a worthwhile risk.

You might enjoy it or not but do your best to get into it gently. Don't be desperate!

Step 5:
Kiss and caress:
Sharing a kiss is the first step toward establishing a physical connection.

A passionate kiss may undoubtedly set a woman up for more, since most women like sharing kisses.

Stimulating your partner's erogenous zones by closeness, kissing, stroking, and caressing them can result in more enjoyable sex.

Additionally, it fosters a deeper sense of safety and connection, two feelings that improve one's performance in bed.

To make your lover desire you, touch and kiss them.

This may make the individual feel more at ease in your company by easing any concerns they may have with their body image.

Kissing is a personal and intimate act, and it's important to approach it with respect and communication.

Here's a step-by-step guide:
Keep in mind that these are general suggestions, and individual preferences may vary:

1. Ensure Consent:
- Before initiating a kiss, make sure there is mutual interest and consent.
Pay attention to verbal and non-verbal cues.

2. Create a Comfortable Atmosphere:
- Choose a comfortable and private setting where you both feel at ease. This can help reduce nervousness and make the moment more enjoyable.

3. Maintain Good Hygiene:
- Ensure that you have fresh breath and maintain good oral hygiene. This consideration shows thoughtfulness and respect.

4. Eye Contact:

- Begin with soft eye contact to gauge the other person's interest. It can build anticipation and connection.

5. Move Closer:

- Gradually close the physical distance between you and your partner. You can start by standing or sitting closer to them.

6. Start with Gentle Touch:

- Use your hands to initiate gentle and subtle touches. For example, place your hand on their arm or gently touch their face.

7. Tilt Your Head:

- Tilt your head slightly to avoid collision and create a comfortable angle for the kiss.

8. Soft and Gentle Lips:

- Begin with soft and gentle lip contact. You can start with closed-mouth kisses and gradually introduce more intensity if the moment feels right.

9. Vary the Pressure:
   - Experiment with the pressure of the kiss. You can alternate between softer and firmer kisses based on the mood.

10. Pay Attention to Response:
   - Be attentive to your partner's response. If they seem comfortable and reciprocate, you can continue; if not, it's important to respect their boundaries.

11. Take It Slow:
   - Allow the moment to unfold naturally. Avoid rushing, and enjoy the connection.

12. Communication:
   - After the kiss, communicate openly about the experience. This can help build understanding and connection.

Remember, the key is to be attentive to your partner's cues and be respectful of their comfort level. Every person and every moment is unique, so there's no one-size-fits-all approach to kissing.

Step 6:
Engage in a lot of foreplay:
Here, you have the option of having your lover undress you or taking off your clothing yourself.

An alternative method would be to take off one article of clothes at a time, keeping the procedure mysterious.

The majority of individuals believe that sex is exclusively penetrative when it comes to foreplay. Nonetheless, there is foreplay in the deed. As the name implies, foreplay is the activity you engage in before having the sex game.

It also involves oral sex, kissing, caressing, and stimulating your partner's erogenous zones.

Ensure that you consume plenty of this. Because you may try out different techniques, it's usually the most fun part of the whole sexual encounter.

Male advice:
Women are capable of many orgasms. Please enjoy your wife; she will be grateful to you in many ways and will be in the mood for more.
Women should know that most guys like being touched, so hug him.
Feel his whole body, touch him, and kiss him.
Don't be the only one hogging the joy and don't hold back.

Step 7:
Select the appropriate time:
It's typically mutually sensed when the time is appropriate for intimate sex.
Select the time when your significant other is most eager to go to the next phase. Sometimes a good indicator of whether it's time is to ask the other person if they're ready or if they want more. When you determine that they are prepared, go to the next phase. Find out more about the ideal time of day for a sexual encounter.

Step 8:
Insertion:
This is the most talked-about aspect of sex and is often thought to be the only thing that takes place.

However, nothing could be farther from the reality.

The penis is introduced into the vagina in this phase.

Male advice:
The stretchy organ known as the vagina is located just below a woman's vulva, or exterior lips of her genitalia.

Before you put your penis into her vagina during protected intercourse, make sure you're using a condom.

Many men misalign their penis, looking about with it as they attempt to enter without realizing where the vagina is, which may cause agony for the lady.

To locate the vagina without feeling ashamed, it's a good idea to ask your spouse for assistance.

Step 9:
Making Love:
After the first penetration is over, you may decide how you both feel about having sex. To guarantee that your girlfriend enjoys the most pleasure, men should make sure to insert your penis into her vagina in rhythmic strokes from the hip. It is ineffective in moving your complete body. Above all, pay attention to your body and your partner.
Permit yourself to enjoy yourself, but remember to consider your partner's happiness as well.

Advice for females:
Take the initiative in bed.
When your malefriend moves, move with him.

It may be enjoyable to thrust each other, especially when you're doing it simultaneously.

Let your malefriend know what you enjoy and dislike.

Make sure you give him pleasure as well.

A person who keeps all the pleasure to self is disliked by everyone.

Step 10:
Final seconds:

You will most likely both be in a sense of euphoria after the intercourse has ended or you have reached your climax.

Permit yourself to be in that condition for whatever long is necessary.

Recall that at this point, you have the option of holding hands or just being close to one another.

Take your time and allow your body to return to its natural condition.

Although rushed sexual encounters may sometimes be thrilling, they can also leave you feeling a little empty within.

Men should take note:
At this time, most women like to be hugged or cuddled. Give her something.

Women's advice:
Let your spouse know whether the event was enjoyable. Nothing compares to the ego boost that comes from having a wonderful time in bed.

Step 11:
Concluding:
The post-coital phase may be charming in some situations and uncomfortable in others. Thus, make an effort to put your companion at ease. Give him/her a t-shirt to wear, make small talk, and compliment the experience.
Grinning, you two laugh together.
Perhaps now is the ideal moment to find a lifelong companion or close friend.
So take advantage of the chance.
Make careful to wash up yourself after you're finished.

Men should wash their penis after taking off the condom, while women should wash their vulva and vagina.
Finally, be careful to properly dispose of the condom.
Keep it out of the toilet.
Instead, place it in a garbage covered with paper or tissue.

Chapter Nineteen

Tips To Get Involved In Best Sex

Has your sex life gone stale?
Between kids, work, the economy, and other pressures, steamy sex may seem like a fantasy.
Although there's a place for that too!
Are you ready to turn up the heat again? These tips will help get you in the mood, both physically and mentally.

Make a Date

Scheduling sex might sound too controlling to be much fun, but sometimes planning is in order.
You book time in your calendar to work out and run errands; why not do the same to prioritize sex?
This is important, so you have to make room for it and push it forward.
Reconnecting with your partner as a lover—not roommates or parents—reminds

you why you were attracted to him in the first place.

And once you've made a sex appointment, the anticipation can be almost as titillating as the event itself.

So kick it up a notch by trading racy texts or leaving a sultry voicemail on his cell.

Forget About "Normal"

Surveys show that American women have a wide variety of sexes.

-17% have tried bondage

-20% have used a blindfold

-30% have had anal sex

-62% masturbate (usually three to four times a week)

-40% use vibrators

-14% look at online porn

-70% need clitoral stimulation to slide into home plate

-18% opt for oral sex

Your quirks and predilections aren't so strange, so quit worrying and enjoy.

Leave the Porn Positions to the Pros
There are a lot of ridiculous standards out there about how women should be, look, or act,
Let all that go.
Reality is, men are turned on by you.
Your partner will be aroused by seeing you turned on too.

Lube Up
The right lubricant can make so-so sex great.
There are several types of lube to try, including water- and silicone-based, so experiment to see what works best for you.

As a general rule, avoid anything that warms, cools, or tastes like a fruit roll-up; these can irritate the skin.

Get Squeaky Clean

Use mouthwash and baby wipes.
Keeping everything fresh is just good manners.

Go Fish

Fish oil reduces inflammation, blood pressure, and dangerous LDL cholesterol.
But guess what?
It also helps open up those very small blood vessels down there.
Fish oil boosts the testosterone in your body (yes, women have this hormone, too), so "you notice your arousal more quickly,"
You can get a hefty dose of fish oil by eating salmon, mackerel, lake trout, sardines, or herring twice a week, but it may be easier to take supplements.

Trade Pain for Pleasure

Sex should feel amazing.

If it's painful, you need to figure out why.

It may be a simple matter of changing positions or adding lubricant.

But it could also be a yeast infection, an undiagnosed STD, endometriosis, painful bladder syndrome, vulvodynia, or even cancer.

Don't try to diagnose it on your own; see your gynaecologists.

If you're still hurting and nothing is medically wrong, consider talking with a certified sex therapist.

There can be emotional reasons for painful sex, particularly for women who've been raised in religious households or who've been sexually abused or raped.

Medication Can Hurt Your Libido

Some medications can blunt your sex drive, including antidepressants, blood pressure medications, and even birth control pills.

If you haven't been feeling as frisky as you'd like, talk to your doctor about whether your prescription might be putting the chill on your libido.

You might be able to take a lower dose or switch to a different drug.

Get to Know Yourself

Forget what you see in movies: Only about 30% of women reach orgasm through penetration alone.

That means a whopping 70% of us need hands-on help to cross the finish line.

It's not all up to your partner, share the responsibility and take on pieces of your sexual pleasure.

Touch yourself to bump up the heat, so you can have more—and better—orgasms.

Give Him Direction

He may not want you telling him how to drive, but he'll appreciate direction about what pleases you. Just don't be bossy about it (unless he's into that, of course).

A simple "It drives me wild when you fill in the blank" can work wonders.

If he's still not getting it, take him by the hand and lead him down the path of your pleasure.

Show him specifically where and how (lightly, firmly, slowly, or quickly) you would like to be touched.

The reward?

A bone-shivering orgasm.

Cultivate a Rich Fantasy Life

You've heard it before:

The most important sexual organ is the brain.

So stock it with sexy images to get your motor revved.

"It's one more tool to bring to your play," There's plenty of tasteful stuff out there, so you don't have to expose yourself to something that's going to offend you.

Create a Sexy Space

You want your bedroom to feel like a place for good lovin', not an office or nursery school.

Remodeling isn't required.

Simply clear out the kid toys, put away the work stuff, and add small touches like candles or flowers.

Get Some Comic Relief

Another thing that happens only in movies is sex without gaffes.

In real life, something's bound to go wrong: one of you farts, you pull a muscle, the dog jumps on you, and you fall off the bed.

The only thing you can do, after checking for broken bones, is to laugh and roll with it. Nothing kills the mood like the pressure to have "perfect sex."

Find Birth Control That Works for You

It's impossible to let yourself go if you're worried about getting pregnant.

This is why the best birth control is the one you'll use without fail.

Fortunately, if you do slip up, there's Plan B, an emergency contraception pill that you can use up to 5 days after sex.

"Plan B is a backup for the condom that breaks or the diaphragm that's 20 miles away,"

"It's not recommended as a primary form of contraception."

Get a Handle on Vascular Conditions

Some health problems affect your sexual life. For example, heart disease, arthritis, hypertension, and diabetes "can profoundly affect our sexual health and pleasure.

What's the connection?

Blood flow.

"Sexual arousal is completely dependent on the blood flow to the tiny blood vessels in our genitals, including the clitoris, which gets erect the same way a man's penis does," Anything that impedes the rush of blood to your northern regions can substantially curb your enthusiasm.

Catch Some Zzz's

About 67% of women have trouble sleeping, according to the National Sleep Foundation. And, as many working women know, when you're really tired, you'd simply rather snooze than get busy with your partner.

Get Fit Down There

You've probably heard it before, but there are good reasons why you should do your Kegels:
"Orgasms are your pelvic floor spasming,"
So "if your pelvic floor muscles aren't very strong, you're not going to feel much."
So how do you do Kegels?
Just squeeze the pelvic floor muscles (these are the ones that control urination) for

several seconds and release and relax the muscles for several seconds.
Make it more fun by squeezing them in sync with music while you're driving.
Do several sets of 20 to 30 reps per set daily.

To make sure you're Kegeling correctly, put a mirror between your legs and watch as you squeeze. The perinea—the skin between the anus and vagina – should pull in, almost like someone's pulling that skin into your body.

Take a Pilates Class
Why Pilates and not another type of exercise?
"Pilates works a lot of ancillary pelvic floor muscles, like the transverse, or higher, abdominal muscles,
Working your transverse abdominals will strengthen your pelvic floor muscles too, similar to what Kegels accomplish.

How sexually adventurous are you?

Would you or could you do it in a park? How about in a car? Some women prefer their sex straightforward, while others aren't satisfied unless they're swinging from the chandeliers.

There's nothing stopping you from catching up with all the pleasure you desire, date it.

Chapter Twenty

Sexual Afterglow

Afterglow simply means a glow remaining where a light has disappeared.

A pleasant effect or feeling that lingers after something is done, experienced, or achieved.

Sexual afterglow refers to the positive emotional and physical sensations that can persist after sexual activity.

It often involves a sense of satisfaction from intimacy and connection between partners.

This period of heightened emotional closeness and contentment can last for varying durations after sexual experiences.

How Much Time Does It Take To Feel Satisfied After A Sex?

Studies have shown that having sex typically improves people's moods; endorphins and other feel-good chemicals are responsible for this.

According to recent research, the benefits of sexual satisfaction could continue for up to two days, and over time, considering partners involved.
Such favorable emotions strengthen relationships between partners.

The researchers examined information from two groups of couples who participated in a two-week diary research study.
There were 96 couples in one sample and 118 couples in the other.
Nearly all of the participants were heterosexual; all were in their first marriages, and none had been married for more than four months.
Every participant filled out a daily survey asking about their level of sexual satisfaction and marital satisfaction, in addition to whether or not they had sex that day.

Couples had an average of four sex encounters throughout the study's 14 days; some did not have any, while others had sex every day. It was discovered that on the day of the encounter, having sex was associated with higher levels of sexual pleasure.

On the other hand, sex also indicated pleasure in the days that followed. In particular, having sex was linked to greater satisfaction levels for the next two days, but it did not predict contentment for the third or longer day.
This indicates that the post-sex increase in sexual pleasure, or the "sexual afterglow," seems to linger for around 48 hours.

The study published that people with a stronger sexual afterglow, that is, people who experienced a higher level of sexual satisfaction will require about 48 hours for another urgent sexual urge to arise.

It was said that forty-eight hours is about equivalent to the duration needed for:
- Optimal conception,
- The restoration of peak sperm concentrations, and
- The maximum viability of sperm in the female reproductive tract.

Sex afterglow, for example, has lingering cognitive implications that last for the same amount of time as the biological implications of sex, which is interesting.

According to the researchers, the study specifically targeted newlyweds, as they have sex more often than long-term couples, which was necessary for the investigation.
In addition, reproduction was the foundation of their theory.
They were a perfect sample to test the predictions since newlyweds are frequently young and of reproductive age.

This explains why young married couples often have sex two to three times a week. This sporadic frequency of sex and its aftereffects might contribute to preserving the highest possible degree of enjoyment.

Thus, why does the afterglow effect happen, and what produces it?

The researchers think it has to do with biological changes that happen during sex, including the release of certain hormones and neurotransmitters (specifically, oxytocin and dopamine).

It is believed that these brain chemicals momentarily increase feelings of contentment.

In turn, this surge is considered adaptive since it fosters the kind of closeness that keeps a partnership going strong.

Some evidence for this theory came from a follow-up poll conducted a few months later, in which the individuals who had the greatest afterglows also reported the highest levels of sexual satisfaction and contentment.

The fact that the researchers were able to duplicate the same pattern of effects in two distinct samples is a significant strength of this study, yet there are several significant limitations.

The research provided evidence for the existence of a sexual afterglow and insight into the average duration of its effects.

Sexual afterglow, is the positive feelings and intimacy experienced after a sexual activity between sexual partners in a relationship.
Also referred to as the satisfaction that lingers after a sexual experience.

Benefits Includes:
1: It does contribute to emotional bonding,
2: It improves mood,
3: It reduces stress,

4: It betters and promotes overall well-being.

5: It increases intimacy

6: It enhances communication between partners,

7: It fosters a stronger connection in the relationship.

Additionally,
This emotional connection from sexual afterglow can contribute to a more fulfilling and positive sexual relationship and a blissful romantic relationship.

Conclusion

Sexual satisfaction is the fulfilment and contentment one experiences in their sexual life regarding a sexual relationship.
It involves a sense of pleasure, intimacy, and emotional well-being derived from sexual activities in a relationship.

Factors contributing to sexual satisfaction can include communication, mutual consent, physical pleasure, emotional connection, and overall relationship dynamics.
Satisfaction varies among individuals and may involve different aspects of the sexual experience.

Benefits Of Sexual Satisfaction

1. Improved Mental Health: Sexual satisfaction is linked to the release of

endorphins and other neurochemicals, contributing to reduced stress and anxiety, and an overall positive impact on mental well-being.

2. Enhanced Relationship Quality: Couples experiencing sexual satisfaction often report higher relationship satisfaction. It fosters emotional intimacy, communication, and a sense of connection between partners.

3. Physical Health: Regular sexual activity can have physical health benefits, such as improved cardiovascular health, better immune function, and even pain relief through the release of natural painkillers.

4. Quality of Sleep: Sexual satisfaction may contribute to better sleep quality, as it can promote relaxation and the release of sleep-inducing hormones.

5. Boosted Self-Esteem: Positive sexual experiences can contribute to increased self-esteem and body

confidence, fostering a positive self-image.
   6. Stress Reduction: Sexual satisfaction has been linked to lower stress levels. Engaging in sexual activities can act as a natural stress-reliever.
   7. Longevity of Relationships: Couples who are sexually satisfied are often more likely to stay together, contributing to the longevity and stability of relationships.

It's important to note that individual experiences may vary, and communication within a relationship is key to understanding and meeting each partner's needs for sexual satisfaction.

Negative Effects Of Sexual Satisfaction

It's important to clarify that sexual satisfaction itself is generally associated with positive effects. However, issues related to sex or relationships can have negative impacts. Here are potential negative effects or challenges related to sexual satisfaction:

1. Mismatched Expectations: If there's a significant disparity in sexual desires or preferences between partners, it can lead to frustration, dissatisfaction, and potentially strain the relationship.
2. Performance Pressure: Feelings of inadequacy or performance pressure can arise, impacting self-esteem and causing anxiety, particularly if individuals feel they are not meeting perceived expectations.
3. Communication Barriers: Lack of open communication about sexual needs, desires, or concerns can lead to misunderstandings, dissatisfaction, and potential relationship issues.
4. Health Concerns: Physical health issues, medications, or hormonal changes can affect sexual satisfaction negatively. Seeking medical advice

may be necessary to address underlying health issues.
5. Emotional Disconnect: If emotional intimacy is lacking, sexual satisfaction may not be fulfilling. Emotional connection and communication are crucial for a satisfying sexual relationship.
6. Relationship Strain: Unresolved conflicts or issues outside the bedroom can spill over into the sexual aspect of a relationship, leading to dissatisfaction and strain.

It's essential for individuals and couples to openly communicate, address any concerns, and seek professional advice if needed to maintain a healthy and satisfying sexual relationship.

In addition to health benefits, sex has
many disadvantages too.
Be knowledgeable before trying it!

Understanding Sexual Satisfaction is
the key to enjoy sexual intercourse in
a romantic relationship.

Don't try sexual adventures until you are of the age that takes responsibility.

How To Achieve Sexual Healing
In Any Relationship is now before you, sign up and get involved for it's possible and achievable.

Enjoy!
Dr. C Conquer